# BEST
# IN
# BEAUTY

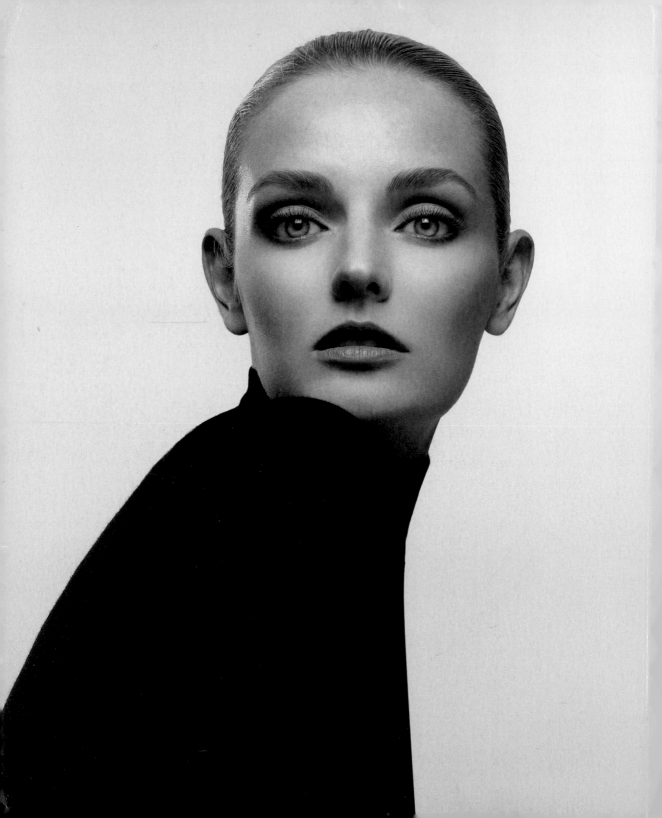

# BEST IN BEAUTY

## AN ULTIMATE GUIDE TO MAKEUP AND SKIN CARE TECHNIQUES, TOOLS, AND PRODUCTS

## RIKU CAMPO

**ATRIA** PAPERBACK

NEW YORK  LONDON  TORONTO  SYDNEY

**ATRIA** PAPERBACK
A Division of Simon & Schuster, Inc.
1230 Avenue of the Americas
New York, NY 10020

First Atria Paperback edition August 2010

**ATRIA** PAPERBACK and colophon are trademarks of
Simon & Schuster, Inc.

For information about special discounts for bulk purchases, please contact
Simon & Schuster Special Sales at
1-866-506-1949 or business@simonandschuster.com.

The Simon & Schuster Speakers Bureau can bring authors to your
live event. For more information or to book an event, contact the
Simon & Schuster Speakers Bureau at 1-866-248-3049 or visit our website
at www.simonspeakers.com.

Designed by Ann Y. Song

Manufactured in the United States of America

10  9  8  7  6  5  4  3  2  1

Library of Congress Cataloging-in-Publication Data
Campo, Riku.
   The best in beauty : an ultimate guide to makeup and skin care
techniques, tools, and products / Riku Campo.—1st Atria paperback ed.
       p. cm.
(ebk)
   1. Beauty, Personal. 2. Feminine beauty (Aesthetics) 3. Beauty culture.
4. Cosmetics. I. Title.
   HQ1219.C36 2010
   646.7'042—dc22

                                                        2010004539

ISBN 978-1-4391-4825-9
ISBN 978-1-4391-5585-1 (ebook)

PHOTO: KURT ISWARIENKO/MODEL: SHANNEN DOHERTY/HAIR: JOHN RUGGIERO/STYLING: EMMA TRASK

This book is dedicated to all beauty junkies who love to play with cosmetics and simply can't live without them. Welcome to my world of beauty.  Best, RIKU

# TABLE OF CONTENTS

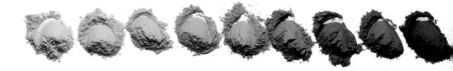

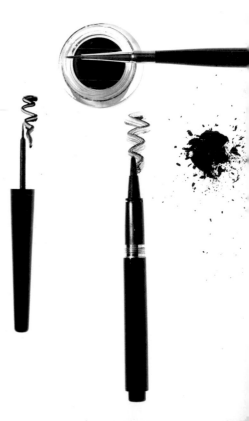

STILL LIFE. KIINO VILLAND

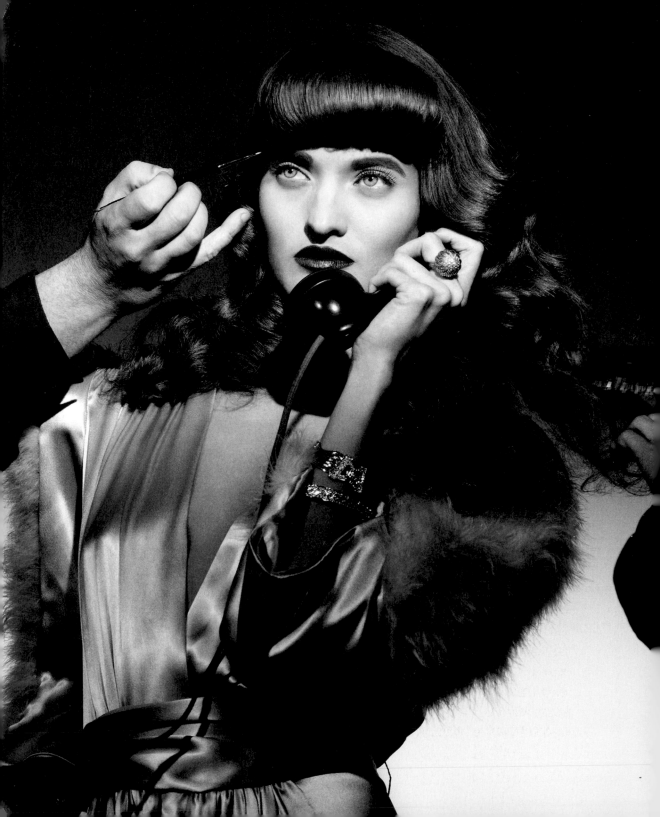

# BEHIND THE SCENES

For as long as I can remember, I have been interested in beautiful things; beautiful clothes, flowers, furniture, buildings, hairdos, fabrics, music, paintings, and then . . . beautiful makeup.

At age nine, I treated my classmates to makeovers in the girls' washroom with the help of colored chalks. And my sister's Barbie dolls got new makeup and hairdos every day. I also cut my friend Rose's long golden locks with big kitchen scissors, but that didn't make her mother happy at all. I was different, and many times I felt like an alien. I studied figure skating and ballet and realized early on that I was a little different from the other boys (who played ice hockey). But colored chalks and my best girlfriends gave me hope that someday I could pursue my passion: makeup!

My mother remembers my telling her at age seven, in 1977, that I wanted to move to Hollywood. Twenty-six years later, I did just that. After high school, though, I attended the only beauty school at the time in Helsinki, Finland. It was 1988, and everything was about heavy pancake foundation, red lips, purple eye shadow, and heavy fuchsia blush. Very '80s. I started questioning the look by using smaller amounts of foundation and powder, using lip gloss on the eyelids, and mixing my own lipsticks using nude eye shadows and Vaseline (I still do that).

That didn't make my teachers very happy, so I quit the beauty school. I knew that makeup could be done many ways, not just one way. The very next day I was hired by Stendahl, the French cosmetic line, as a demonstration makeup artist at the biggest department store in Finland. There was always a long line at my makeup chair, and I was the only male makeup artist in town at the time. For the next two years I did hundreds of faces a day. The amazing '80s looks were good in MTV music videos but not necessarily in harsh daylight. And especially not in Finland in the middle of the winter, when the light is gray and, well, not so flattering.

Though having your makeup done by a professional is a great treat, I learned that women are more comfortable with makeup they can easily do themselves. They don't want to spend more than ten minutes applying it every morning. Or three minutes. Otherwise, they'd rather not wear makeup at all. The '80s makeup idea was all about transformations, and now it is all about being yourself, with a little help from cosmetics. A couple of years later came grunge, which revolutionized the whole fashion and beauty industry; everything became more relaxed, street, and natural. My motto, "Less is more," seemed to work well for this new generation. Kate Moss, Kristen McMenamy, Johnny Depp, and Marky Mark were the new fashion idols, and the no-makeup look was the "it" thing all over the world.

When I finally settled in Los Angeles in 2003, I was blinded by the beautiful California nature. Very soon I noticed the American way of feminine beauty and its countless variations: so many beautiful skin colors and mixes opened my eyes to this nation. I had the luck to work with a cosmetic company that flew me all over the United States. In two months I saw more than twenty states. It was a wonderful experience, not only because I love traveling but also because I met so many women with so many different skin colors. I realized that there are regional differences in makeup styles, the same kind of variations you can see in Europe (southern Europeans wear more makeup than do central and northern Europeans). Europe and America are distinct in that Americans take eyebrow grooming more seriously than their European counterparts do. Almost everyone here has beautifully groomed eyebrows. The other difference is nail care: manicures and pedicures are very common in the United States, but in Europe they are pure luxury and quite expensive. And then there's the hair: Americans always have very beautiful, healthy, and feminine hairstyles (most Europeans love shorter, more bohemian, practical styles).

California is all about the sun and beach. Skin care is more important than makeup. California ladies wear just SPF or tinted moisturizer with SPF, mascara, pink peach blush or bronzer, and lip gloss—sometimes not even that. Very relaxed. East Coast ladies are more specific with their looks, wearing more serious makeup. I see this especially in the use of lipsticks: their lips are lined very carefully, and the whole look is very well put together: makeup, hair, and clothes—very businesslike. You can see the perfect liquid eyeliner with those 1950s wings, and perfectly lined true red lips. Or maybe the most sophisticated nude matte makeup. In Miami it's much more makeup in the celebration of colors; cool tones meet warm tones and everything in between. Compared to California, it's quite the opposite—surprisingly.

Chicago's style seems to be very close to that of the East Coast but also takes into account the cold winter winds and rains and the humid summer weather. Such severe weather conditions are challenging for makeup and skin care. Texas is all about femininity; the ladies love to do makeup and bigger hairdos. That is no cliché; the southern belle is alive and well! It is applause for being a woman! This is the motto in all the southern states that I have visited and worked in. It's almost that early '90s style with the perfect, strong makeup look. Fun and exciting!

As a makeup artist, I have many beauty icons who inspire me to mix new and old looks. We all love Hollywood legends because of their glam looks, and so do I—especially silent movie stars. In the 1980s I loved the looks of the model Tania Coleridge, who starred in George Michael's video "Father Figure," as well as the singer Corinne Drewery of Swing Out Sister. I guess it was the bob-hairdo and red-lips combination that fascinated me as an artist. And I don't think I was the only gay boy who loved those looks! But my real inspiration has been two singers whose music and lyrics have been epochal in my career: Kate Bush and the Italian singer Alice. Yes, music and art can also be an inspiration for a makeup artist. It's all visual!

Cubism opened my eyes to art (the early Cubism of 1907–1911 is my favorite period). I really like the way the artists painted at that time. I admire Sonia Delaunay, who also designed textiles and set and costume designs for theater productions in Paris, France. The self-portraits of the Finnish painter Helene Schjerfbeck (1862–1946) also had a big influence on me. I remember staring at her works in art books when I was a little boy and wondering how she had captured that fragile, beautiful look. It was very touching for me. It still is. Beauty never dies.

You can emphasize your beauty with the right makeup. And you don't need to change into something different to be a beauty. All you need is confidence and fun.

It is not a serious game. At the end of the day, you will wash it off your face and try something new.

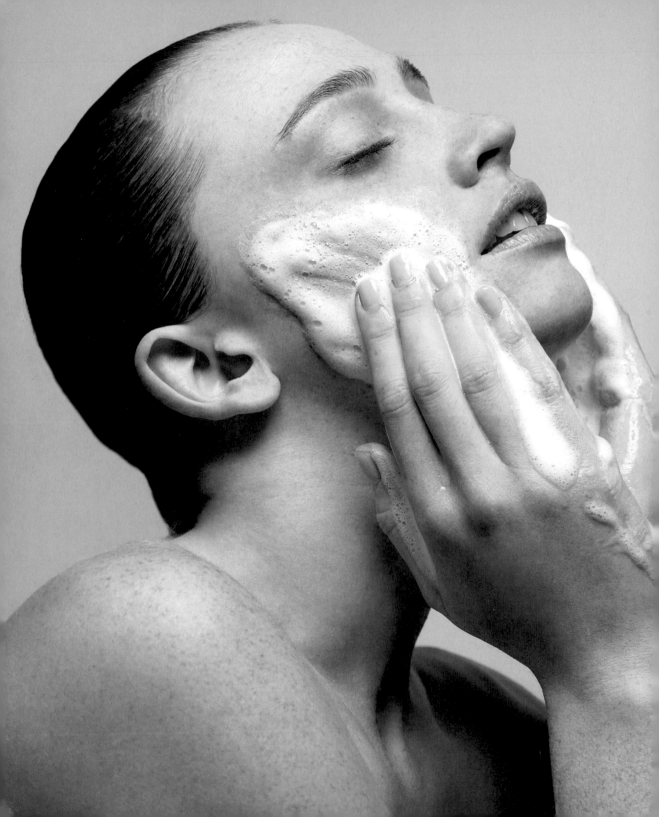

# 1 FACIAL CARE

**Ole Henriksen** *Skin Care guru, Esthetician, and Spa Owner*

When I moved to Los Angeles, I looked for a good esthetician with whom I could build a relationship and who would help solve my dry-skin problem. I had read an article about Ole Henriksen Spa in a beauty magazine in the early 1990s in which there was a beautiful photo of him and the British actress Patsy Kensit.

PHOTO: PASCAL DEMEESTER/MODEL: JODIE/HAIR: KEIKO HAMAGUCHI/NAILS: BETH FRICKE

I sought out Ole, who instantly made an impression on me. He is one of the most positive people I've ever encountered. His energy was just so high. There was such an aura around him, an aura of pure happiness and joy. I thought he was the best walking advertisement of his profession!

Ole introduced me to Maki, who has been the miracle worker on my skin. And now, after five years of being a client of Ole's spa, not only does my skin look ten times better (no dry areas or flakes or one single milium), this Danish-born skin genius has also become my friend.

Here is what Ole says about skin care:

A professional esthetician is the best person to determine your skin type and its condition, but you can also analyze your skin yourself. This analysis will help you become your own skin care expert, allowing you to focus on treatment methods to elevate your skin to its best.

## HOW TO ANALYZE YOUR SKIN

Three Things Needed to Analyze Your Skin Correctly

1. Bright daylight, as skin reveals itself best in this light
2. A large-handled mirror, ideally 25 centimeters or bigger in diameter
3. Your own beautiful face, free of makeup

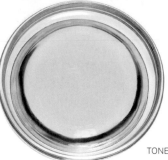

TONERS FOR DRY, COMBINATION, AND OILY SKIN.

**STEP 1**

Take an inventory of your skin. The focus should be on texture, muscle tone, hydration, pigmentation, pores, and capillary strength.

**STEP 2**

Glide your hand across the four primary parts of your face: forehead, nose, cheeks, and chin.

*How is your skin texture?* Soft, smooth, or slightly coarse in areas, with occasional bumpiness?

*How is your skin muscle tone?* Firm, with defined facial contours, or less-defined facial contours, showing signs of loosening, especially in the lower parts of the face and neckline?

*Do you have fine expression lines or wrinkles?*
How is the skin around your eyes? Taut, or is there some wrinkle formation?
Are you prone to fluid retention under your eyes?

*How is your skin hydration level?* Excessive and therefore oily, or dehydrated and therefore dry, or a combination?

*How is the pigmentation of your skin?* Perfectly uniform? Uneven in some facial zones, with brown spots or white spots, which signify pigment loss?

*How are the pores in your skin?* Mostly tight and invisible, which typifies dry skin, or more open and visible in the center of your face, which typifies oily skin?

*How strong are the capillaries in your skin?* This is basically signified by the number of visible capillaries. Frail capillaries typically show as redness, particularly in the cheeks, which indicates greater sensitivity to the elements and therefore sensitive skin. The right treatments can gradually strengthen the facial capillaries.

## THE BASIC SKIN TYPES

The basic skin types are dry, oily, and combination. Most normal skin has both dry and oily parts, which makes it combination. That's why I label my products for dry, oily, or normal/combination skin. Sensitive skin can be experienced by all skin types and age brackets.

### DRY SKIN: BASIC FACTS

- 60 percent of skin is dry.
- Dry skin is the closest thing to normal skin.
- Dry skin is more common with fair skin than with darker skin.
- When you pinch dry skin, it turns red.
- Cold weather, too much showering, and air-conditioning in the winter are not good for dry skin; the skin might turn even drier, and flaky.
- Dry skin is often sensitive or has sensitive areas, such as the eyelids, cheeks, and forehead.
- Drinking six to eight glasses of purified water a day is the best way to moisturize the skin from the inside out, all year round.

### OILY SKIN: BASIC FACTS

- This skin type is predominantly oily, or at least 60 percent of its surface is. The T-zone is where the pores produce the most oil and pores tend toward blackhead formation. Sometimes these blackheads become inflamed and turn into pus-filled pimples.
- Shiny skin is a frequent problem for people with oily skin. With the right care, based on purifying and antiseptic extracts, this skin type can be stabilized, resulting in tighter pores, fewer eruptions, and less shiny skin.

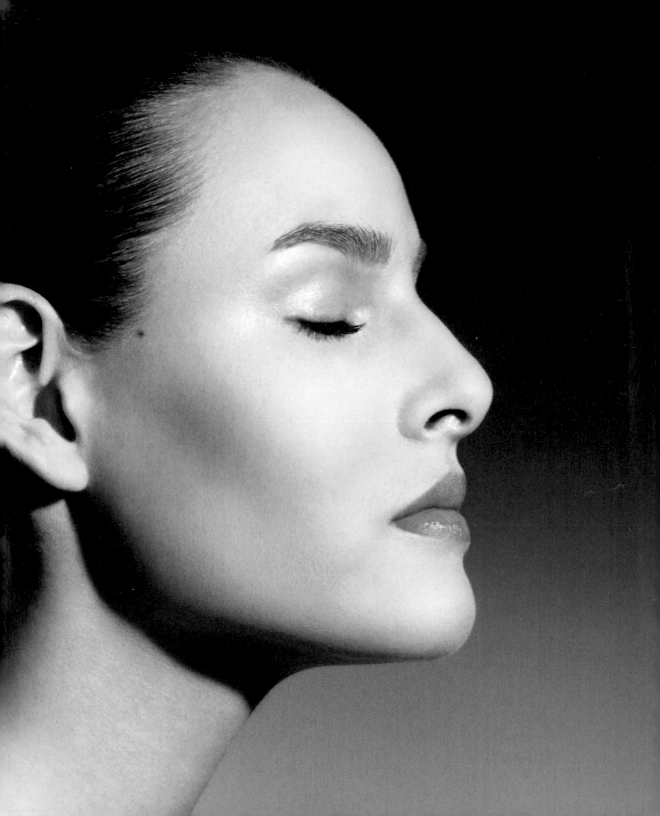

- Sebum, produced by the sebaceous glands, is a natural skin lubricant. When produced in balanced proportions, it adds natural softness and protection to the skin, but when overproduced, as in oily or acneic skin, it causes clogged pores and possibly inflammation. So it can be a friend or an enemy of your skin.

- Heredity, diet, and hormones (oily skin is more common, for example, among teenagers) can all cause skin to turn oily, but skin can also turn oily in later years due to bodily imbalances or the use of products that are too greasy. Extremely humid weather also contributes to making the oil and sebaceous glands even more active, which makes the skin look shiny and greasy.

- Blackheads and whiteheads are common problems in oily skin, but you can get rid of them by using my A.M. and P.M. cleansing routine, focused on dislodging the pores of dirt and grime, including even the most stubborn pore clogging. But don't squeeze your pores; you might get rid of some of the blackheads or whiteheads, but if they are not eliminated properly (which can easily happen), bacteria will form in the pores and you will reinfect them, resulting in even more inflamed blemishes. Leave that kind of treatment to a professional esthetician or dermatologist, who will do a proper job of deep cleaning the skin. Try to go one to two times monthly to make rapid progress.

- It is not a myth that people with oily skin don't get wrinkles as easily as people with dry skin; oily skin remains more flexible and resilient because of all the oil. Darker skin tends to be more oily than fair skin because darker skin has larger oil glands than fair skin does.

## COMBINATION SKIN: BASIC FACTS

- Combination skin means that some parts of your face are oily and typically have visible pores, mostly on the nose and cheeks, while the rest of the face is anywhere from normal to dry.

- Seasonal changes frequently cause changes in combination skin: in the summer it becomes oilier and more prone to blackhead and whitehead formation in the T-zone, while the winter season causes it to become drier, especially in the cheek area.

## SKIN CARE ROUTINES, BY SKIN TYPE

A simple daily morning and night skin care regimen should focus on:

Cleaning

Hydrating

Sun protection

Antiaging serums and peeling/exfoliating products

### A.M. AND P.M. SKIN CARE ROUTINE FOR DRY SKIN

**A.M.: The focus should be on protecting the skin from the elements.**

1. Cleanse with a gentle, water-rinseable cleansing lotion or foam.
2. Tone with a spray tonic with antioxidants. It's a great wake-up call for the skin and feels very refreshing.
3. Day cream is all about hydration and sun protection, so use one with SPF 15. When at sunny resorts, use SPF 30.
4. Finally, on the eyes use a richly textured eye cream. A dense eye cream will create greater resiliency in the delicate under-eye tissue, so that the skin will be less prone to wrinkle formation due to typical facial expressions.

**P.M.: The focus should be on antiaging and repair.**

1. Cleanse as in the morning. Do a double cleansing if you're wearing a foundation.
2. Tone with a spray tonic.
3. Use facial serum for antiaging and repair. Look for one with a high concentration of antioxidants.
4. Use a night cream with a rich texture, ideally based on peptides for firming and natural acids for cell proliferation.
5. Use an eye gel for firming and recontouring the lid and under-eye region. Keep it in the fridge for extra cooling, antipuffiness, and firming benefits.

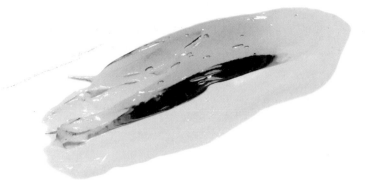

## Once a Week

1. Fill your bathroom sink one-third full of warm water, and pour 10 to 15 drops of lavender essential oil into it. Drench a terry facecloth in the aromatic water and press it firmly onto your face. Hold in place for about 30 seconds while taking in the purifying, calming, and uplifting benefits of the essential oil. Repeat five to eight times. This delicious treat prepares the skin for exfoliation.

2. Exfoliate with a gentle scrub. Massage the scrub into the skin with tiny circular motions for two to three minutes. Rinse with lukewarm water.

3. Hydrate, nourish, and renew your skin with a hydrating mask. Don't forget to apply it on the neck as well. Lie down and relax for 10 to 15 minutes while the active ingredients of the mask go to work. Rinse with lukewarm water.

4. Follow with serum, night cream, and eye gel. Eye-area cream is so important. It isn't enough to use your regular day or night cream around the eyes because there are no oil glands in the skin surrounding them. That means no natural lubricants protect this highly expressive part of the face. The skin under the eyes is also very thin and sensitive, so I can't overemphasize the importance of using a richly textured eye cream or gel. A richly textured eye cream will literally form a protective barrier over the skin in this region, providing both enhanced elasticity and comfort. Eye gels are also great at reducing puffiness under the eyes, especially if formulated with ingredients such as cucumber extract. The reason that your day or night cream isn't enough is the higher

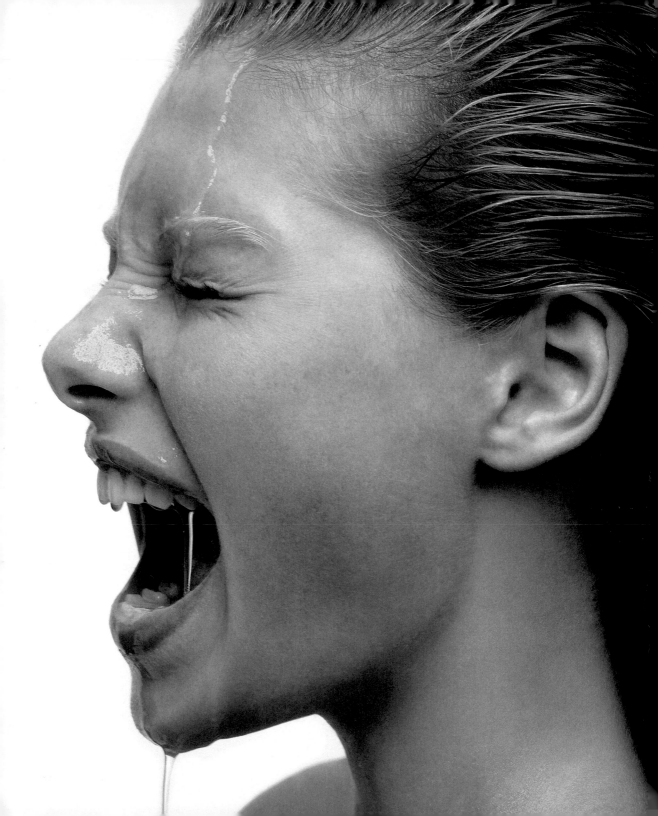

concentration of water-based ingredients in these formulations, which can cause them to slip into the eyes and put a foggy mantle over them.

## A.M. AND P.M. SKIN CARE ROUTINE FOR OILY SKIN

Cleanse twice a day with a soothing, nondrying antiseptic gel or foam cleanser, ideally containing eucalyptus or tea tree essential oils. Don't wash more than twice a day, because washing excessively will cause the oil and sebaceous glands to produce more oil, especially if too much oil is stripped away in the cleansing process. Use a flat round vegetable sponge to activate the cleanser and glide it across the skin in a light circular motion, covering every little crevice of the face and neck. On any part of the face afflicted with infected blemishes such as pimples and cysts, avoid using the sponge since it can be irritating on this very sensitive tissue. The second step is the application of a disinfecting and pore-constricting skin tonic based, ideally, on camphor and lactic acid. Apply with a cotton pad, stroking across the entire face in a gentle manner.

### A.M.

1. Cleanse and tone as described above.
2. Apply medicated blemish gel as a day cream if your skin is erupted in the T-zone. For oily skin with no blemishes, use an oil-free moisturizer based on cell-proliferating extracts such as sugar maple, sugarcane, and lemon peel extracts.
3. Finally, apply an eye gel.

### P.M.

1. Cleanse and tone as in the morning.
2. Apply a medicated potion, contained in a roll-on blemish stick, on the areas where eruptions are a problem.
3. Apply a night gel based on calming and pore-refining algae and cell-renewing fruit acid extracts, which also purify the skin.
4. Apply eye gel.

**Two to Three Times a Week**

1. Exfoliation is one of the most important skin care routines for oily skin, because it cleanses the clogged pores and washes away dead skin cells. You should do this every other day and follow your regular skin care routine afterward.

2. Use a pore-refining clay or mud mask that removes impurities twice a week. Leave the mask on the skin until it is totally dry, then rinse it off with cool water. Cool water keeps the pores closed, while warm water opens them up (you don't want to open the pores after you just closed them with the mask).

## A.M. AND P.M. SKIN CARE ROUTINE FOR COMBINATION SKIN

**A.M.: The focus should be on protecting the skin against the elements.**
You want to establish balance so that the skin doesn't look excessively oily in the T-zone as the day progresses, especially during the summer.

1. Cleanse with a foaming gel cleanser, activated with a flat, round complexion sponge. The sponge will gently exfoliate and deep clean your skin.
2. Tone with a spray tonic based on pore-constricting extracts.
3. Hydrate with a light-textured day cream based on soothing and balancing extracts.
4. Finally, apply eye cream—a richly textured formulation including essential fatty acids from vegetable sources.

**P.M.: The focus should be on antiaging and repair.**

1. Cleanse as in the morning.
2. Tone as in the morning.
3. Use an oil-free serum in a gel base. Look for one with both antiaging and antiseptic benefits.
4. Use a light-textured night cream, based on cell-renewing and pore-tightening ingredients.
5. Use an eye gel or cream for under-eye protection and firming.

## Once a Week

Do the same routine as described under dry skin, on p. 11.

*What is a skin toner, and what are the benefits of using one?*

A skin toner or tonic used immediately after a cleanser acts as an all-in-one cell proliferator, pore constricter, and purifier, all of which are important in elevating the skin to be the best it can be. Oily skin, especially if it's prone to clogging and eruptions, will respond well to skin tonics with ingredients such as goldenseal, camphor, and lactic acid from milk. Skin tonics infused with fruit and berry extracts are particularly beneficial for dry and combination skin. Apply skin tonic to a premoistened flat, round cotton pad and gently press the pad into the skin. Pressing the tonic into the skin rather than rubbing it on ensures greater absorption of the active ingredients.

Wash in the morning with a facial wash, and then use a toner. I highly recommend that a cleanser and toner be used in tandem each morning. A gentle foaming or lotion cleanser used with a flat, round complexion sponge is a great way to polish and awaken the skin and get the circulation going, while a toner, with its many active ingredients, will brighten the overall appearance of the skin. The treatment products that follow, such as serum and moisturizer, will interact much more effectively with the skin after cleanser and toner are used.

*At what age should I start to use antiaging creams?*

You can never start too young with antiaging formulations. Most of us don't think of sunscreens as having antiaging benefits, but they do, by cutting out a great portion of the harmful UVA and UVB rays that cause premature wrinkle formation and sagging of the skin. Antiaging is really about prevention, which includes a healthy diet and exercise.

I have always been a champion of natural beauty and growing old in a natural way. You should never fight the aging process as though it's your enemy but embrace it with the right care, and that way you'll grow old looking absolutely beautiful. Be proud of where you are in your life; each day is a gift, and aging is part of it. The wisdom, inner peace, and confidence gained with each passing year are priceless. When you remain fit and healthy, with glowing skin texture, you will look stunning at any age!

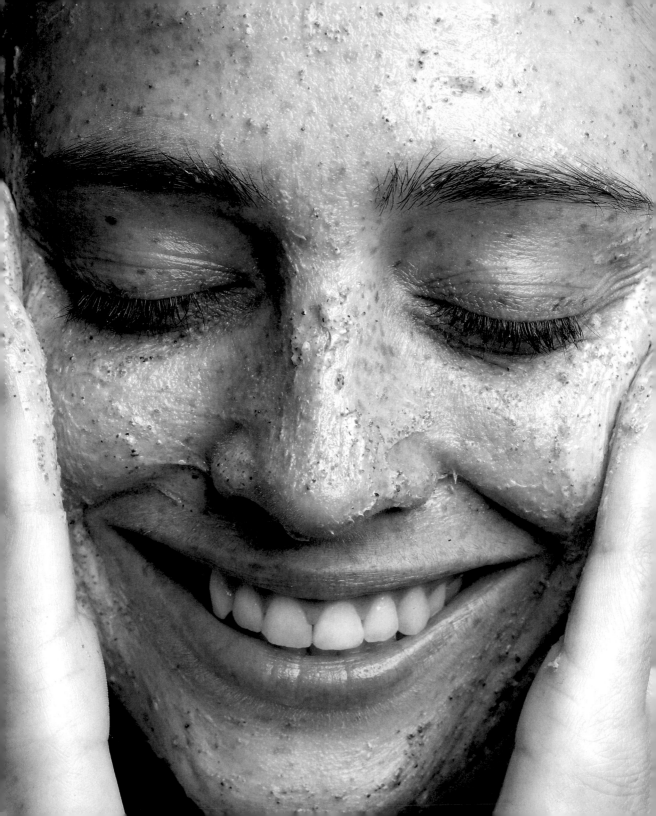

Start each day, regardless of age, by saying to your mirror image, "Good morning, I love myself and I am beautiful." And do it with a big smile!

### What about complexion treatments?

Most people think that professional face treatments don't do anything. You get a great face massage, and your skin is left red and irritated afterward. There's a lot more to a complexion treatment than a facial massage! Everyone should start having complexion treatments beginning at age 16 to 18. They're truly an investment in the future of your skin. The key is to find a fabulous esthetician through a trusted recommendation. A skilled esthetician will know what the best treatment approach for your individual skin should be. Should it be a treatment focused on deep cleansing and pore tightening, or calming and soothing, or lifting and firming, or is a series of microdermabrasions best suited to your skin? A good esthetician should explain every step of the treatment she or he is giving you, what the benefits are, and what you are meant to feel on your skin with the different products used.

A gentle touch applied throughout a treatment is better than a heavy touch, so look for that. However, a deep-cleansing complexion treatment can leave the skin slightly red if there are a lot of clogged pores to be dealt with. If the elimination of the impurities is done correctly, the redness will subside within 24 hours.

### How do I know if I have used the wrong skin care products on my face?

You can tell if, for instance, you have used a dry-skin day cream on your oily skin, or vice versa. Since oily skin often has more visible pores and may be prone to erupting, a cream formulated for dry skin used on this skin type can spell trouble. Because of the richer and more emollient extracts in this kind of day cream, oily skin will experience more clogged pores and inflamed blemishes, such as pimples. Using a cream formulated for oily skin on dry skin will create less of a problem, except that this skin type will feel less smooth to the touch and look duller, due to lack of adequate hydration.

### How can I prevent and address skin problems?

Both women and men can experience skin problems. To achieve the best skin possible, first remember that skin is a living, breathing organ with amazing powers of renewal. The top layer of the skin, known as the stratum corneum, is constantly undergoing renewal via the shedding of dead skin cells. A new top layer of skin is created approximately every 25 to 30 days. In young skin the renewal cycle is more frequent than in older skin. As new skin is constantly forming from below, there is always room to improve the appearance of the skin by using the right products and treatment methods. Even the most problematic skin can be elevated to a level of perfection that you may never have thought possible.

### What are cysts?

Cysts are red lumps underneath the skin's surface that are often painful. They look like small swellings. They don't form a head with visible pus, as pimples do. A word to the wise: resist the temptation to squeeze cysts and pimples. Doing so will prolong their presence by weeks. Rather, use an antiblemish product twice a day, evening and morning, for three to six days, and the cyst or pimple should disappear.

### What is microdermabrasion?

Microdermabrasion, which is done by a professional, polishes, exfoliates, and oxygenates the skin, repairing the damage done by too much sun. The treatments also attack fine wrinkles, gradually making them less visible. Skin with fine acne scars will also see amazing improvements from a series of at least six treatments. I was the first person to introduce microdermabrasion to the West Coast many years ago, and I benefit from this treatment myself. Many celebrities flock to my spa before red-carpet events for this truly results-driven treatment.

Microdermabrasion is not good for all skin types, though. If you have sensitive skin or a lot of blemishes, it is not the best solution.

### What can I do about enlarged pores?

You can improve the texture of your skin by using an energizing complexion scrub three times a week and a tightening clay-based firming mask once a week.

# Dr. Douglas Hamilton,
## UCLA professor and dermatologist

*When your skin problems are severe, turn to a dermatologist, a doctor who can analyze the condition of your skin and design a healing treatment.*

*Cosmetic dermatology is a specialty concerned with treating acne scars, wrinkles, and cellulite. For example, chemical peels; laser treatments (such as $CO_2$ laser and N-Lite); wrinkle-filling treatments such as Botox (for forehead and crows' feet at the corners of the eyes); Restylane, and Juvéderm (fillers for smile lines); and the nonsurgical face-lift called Thermage.*

### Chemical Peels
*This is a treatment for the removal of aged skin by the application of a chemical, typically to the face and hands. A "superficial chemical peel" can result in moderate improvement of brown spots, even out irregular skin color, and reduce fine wrinkles. The patient can have the treatment, then return to work the next day. The results last about a year. A "medium peel" yields a greater improvement of aged skin. The patient may need one to two weeks off from work, but the results last several years.*

### Laser Treatments
*Treatments such as $CO_2$ that involve lasers remove the top layer of skin and vaporize the high ridges of wrinkles. This is good for smoothing the surface of wrinkled, blemished, and sun-damaged skin, and it smoothes out acne scars as well.*

### Laser Hair Removal

The laser selectively targets the pigment inside the hair follicle. Each pulse of the laser disables large numbers of hair follicles. The hair doesn't grow back in the areas where hair follicles are killed. You usually need three to six treatments to get results.

Note: Dark skin doesn't respond well to this treatment, which can actually cause dark spots.

### Acne Treatments

There are three main treatment options. Treatment is usually continued for months.

1. Creams/gels: Benzoyl peroxide (this kills the bacteria Cleocin T)
2. Retinoids: Three brands—Tazorac, Differin, and Retin-A—prevent clogging of the pores
3. Pills: Antibiotics, birth control pills, and spironolactone

### Botox

This is one of the most common beauty fillers all over the world. It has been said to be poisonous and cause bad headaches, though it has no proven significant side effects. You will see the results with Botox in about a week.

### Restylane and Juvéderm

Both are used to fill fine lines and wrinkles.

### Thermage

This is a very popular nonsurgical face-lift. A radio-frequency technology is used to heat the layers of your skin; it delivers heat deep into the skin to cause curling (tightening) of existing collagen and stimulate new collagen growth.

Many times you need just one treatment to see the results, depending on your skin condition. A Thermage treatment lasts three to five years.


### Photo Facial Rejuvenation

Intense pulsed light (IPL) is used to treat and correct a variety of skin conditions, such as irregularity of color (brown and red spots), poor skin texture, small veins, enlarged pores, rosacea, and signs of aging due to sun exposure. Three to six treatments yield results. You can return to work the same day and resume all of your regular activities.

Rosacea is a skin ailment that leaves people red-faced from dilated blood vessels and chronic flushing. Photo facial rejuvenation can successfully treat dilated blood vessels and redness without injuring the surrounding healthy skin, while greatly reducing the episodes of flushing with long-term effectiveness.

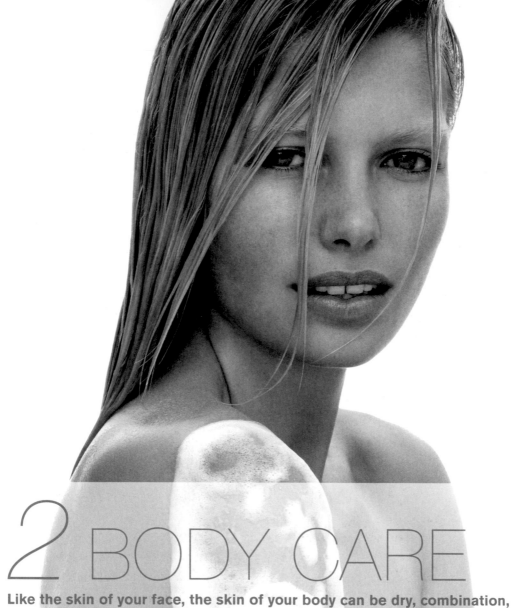

# 2 BODY CARE

Like the skin of your face, the skin of your body can be dry, combination, or oily. The seasons, where you live (in the desert, by the ocean, in the country, or in a big city), your lifestyle, and your genes will all influence how the biggest organ of your body, the skin, feels and looks.

# DAILY CARE
## Dry Skin

Take very quick showers under warm water, never hot, because hot water is drying and can result in rashes. Use a moisturizing body wash that is soap- and fragrance-free. Exfoliate the skin once a week with the mildest body exfoliation cream. After showering, use a body oil, lotion, or cream.

## Oily Skin

Use an antiseptic body wash that will also disinfect the possible blemishes on your back. Use a natural sponge. Exfoliation is also important, to get rid of dead cells. This also deep cleans the pores and makes you feel fresher. You can exfoliate your body every day, but if you have pimples on your back, don't scrub too much. You don't want them to open and get red or infected. Be light-handed. After showering, use an oil-free body moisturizer.

## Sensitive Skin

Use fragrance-free products only.

# EXTRA CARE
## Dry Brushing

Dry brushing your body in small circular motions helps increase blood circulation, tone muscles, and create a sense of well-being.

Begin with small sections: start with the soles of the feet, then do the legs and arms, and finish with the chest and back. Always massage toward the heart. Follow with a warm shower and use a body wash. Blot your body dry and apply body oil or cream or an anticellulite cream. Anticellulite cream doesn't work overnight. Use it twice a day on the desired areas—hips, thighs, and legs—and with the right diet, a lot of exercise, and dry brushing you will see results.

## Massage

A whole-body massage is great for relieving stress and tension, and it can keep your body loose and pain-free and benefit your overall health.

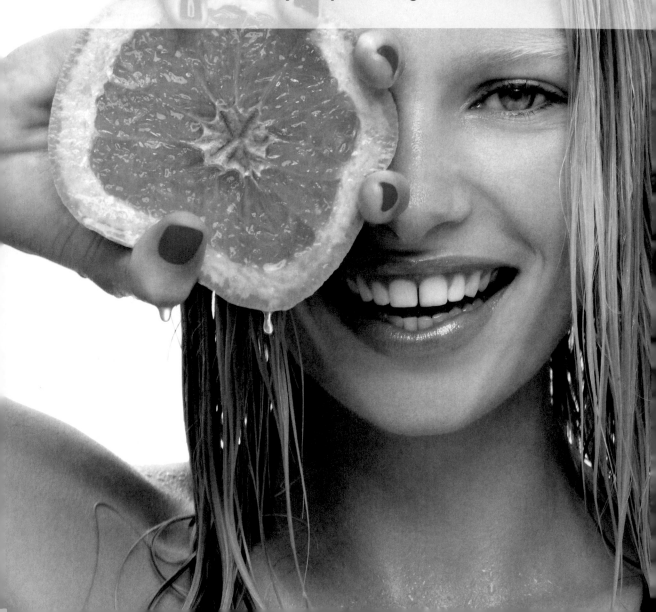

# 3 NUTRITION

**Good nutrition is a key component of great skin care.**

**Debra Santelli,** *nutritionist who specializes in holistic nutrition and healing foods*

## VITAMINS AND MINERALS FOR THE SKIN

Food-based nutrients that help support the skin include bee pollen and propolis, which prevent wrinkles; grapefruit, which improves the complexion; papaya and pineapple; essential fatty acid–containing foods such as fish, flax, and avocado oils, to help improve the visual appearance of the skin; and cucumber, carrot, cabbage, garlic, and ginger juice.

When vitamins and minerals aren't taken in through foods, the skin can suffer and age prematurely. Deficiencies can lead to ailments such as acne, black eyes, dandruff, dermatitis, dry skin, eczema, hives, itching, enlarged pores, skin allergies, stretch marks, and wrinkles.

Good nutrition heals. For example, it can help alleviate or prevent eczema. Beneficial bacteria can be found in probiotics or non-sugared yogurt or kefir. Vitamins such as biotin, inositol, and vitamins A, B2, B6, B12, and C also help eczema. Borage, evening primrose, and various fish, flaxseed, and olive oils can be beneficial in the treatment because they replenish essential fatty acid deficiencies. Hydrochloric acid deficiencies can be an underlying cause of some cases of eczema.

Make sure that your diet is full of a variety of fresh, organic vegetables and fruits. Taking additional vitamins and minerals will only enhance the nutrition you receive from food.

A well-balanced diet, full of fresh organic vegetables, fruits, nonhormone proteins, whole grains, and healthy oils, along with plenty of clean water, is your best ticket to health and beauty.

## WATER

Drink half your weight in ounces for basic hydration each day; this will help prevent constipation, allergies, fatigue, migraines, wrinkles, and acne.

## SUGAR

We hear and read that sugar is like a poison, and then we replace it with an artificial sweetener. If you must use a sweetener, choose stevia, a natural alternative to sugar. But the best way to satisfy a sweet tooth is by eating fresh fruit.

## NAILS AND HAIR

The most important vitamins and minerals to take to keep nails and hair strong, shiny, and healthy-looking are essential fatty acids, a multiple vitamin, calcium, zinc, biotin, and vitamin B12. Make sure there are no underlying health conditions causing hair or nail issues. For example, conditions such as hypothyroidism, adrenal issues, and hormonal imbalances can cause hair and nails to be dry, brittle, and weak.

### See a nutritionist:
- To achieve optimum health
- As you age
- When health challenges arise

# Leslie Bega, Actress

*Leslie is living proof of what a healthy lifestyle, including raw foods and yoga, can do. This is what Leslie says:*

*My daily routines are nonconventional. I work on the inside and let the outside be a reflection of that. You are what you eat.*

*I use skin care products, but they are simple and organic raw, based on seaweed. Seaweed has one of the largest nutritional mineral element contents of all the products on the market.*

*It's important to know what you are putting into and on your body. I am the kind of person who has always read every ingredient label of every product. I drink a lot of water, and I take MSM, which is a sulfur-bearing molecule. It adds permeability and flexibility to the entire cellular structure of your body. It's a beauty and skin nutrient. I also try to incorporate as much raw/living foods into my diet as possible, and I*

PHOTO: PASCAL DEMEESTER/HAIR: KEIKO HAMAGUCHI/SYLING: HEIDI MEEK

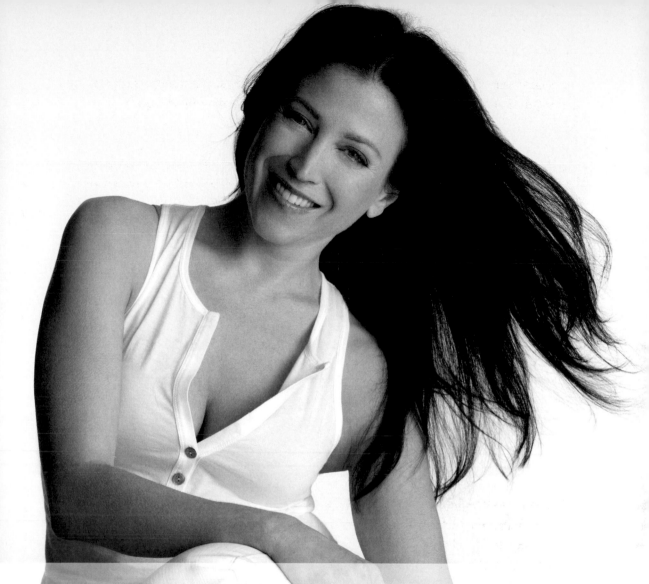

eat everything organic. I helped open the Planet Raw restaurant in Santa Monica, and eating this way is very healthy, as the food preserves all its natural enzymes, vitamins, and nutrients, so your body is receiving whole nutrition. It helps maintain proper brain chemistry, so your system remains more balanced. Interestingly enough, my skin has become more beautiful over the years. Again, it has to do with my diet. I don't wear any foundation anymore, and my skin is clear and glows.

And my beauty trick that works whenever I need a little lift—yoga!

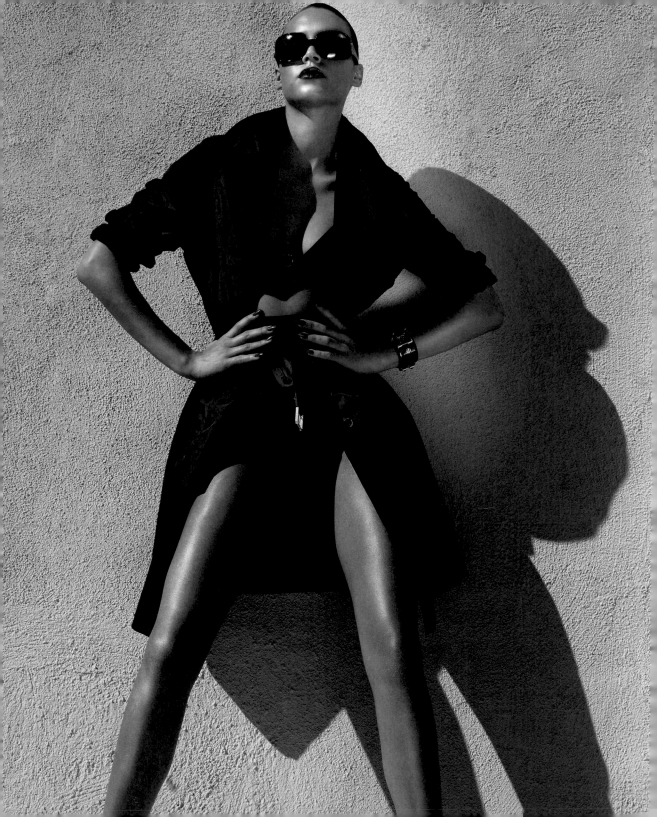

# 4 WAXING

PHOTO: DANIELA FEDERICI/MODEL: ALANA/HAIR: DAMIAN MONZILLO/STYLING: HANI/PUBLISHED AT MADAME, GERMANY

**Lidia Tivichi,** *esthetician and skin specialist at Kimara Ahnert Studio, New York*

Waxing is a semipermanent hair removal process that removes hair from the root. Women commonly remove hair from their legs, eyebrows, upper lip, underarms, and pubic areas. Waxing is also one of the most popular beauty treatments in the United States today.

### How much does waxing cost?
Between $20 to $150, depending on the areas that are being waxed.

## Types of Waxing
- Bikini: Leaves some pubic hair, but takes away most of it
- Brazilian: Takes off all the pubic hair

Note: Don't wax if you have eczema or psoriasis.

# 5 HOME SPA

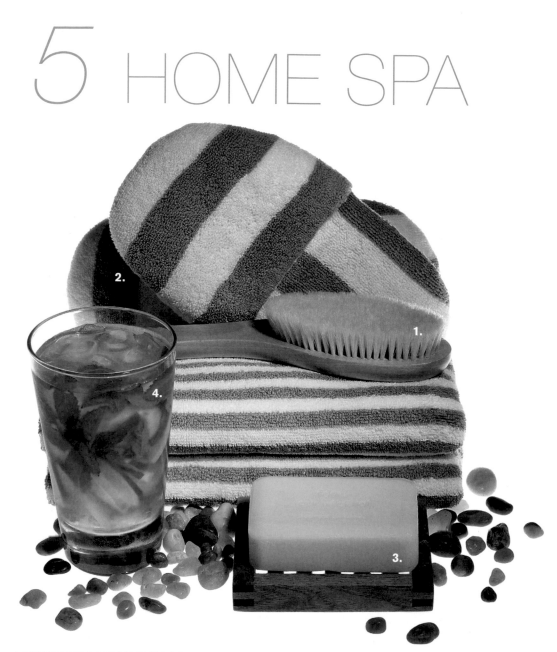

**1.** DRY BRUSH **2.** COMFY SLIPPERS AND A SOFT TOWEL **3.** LIME ESSENTIAL OIL SOAP **4.** LIME, CUCUMBER, AND MINT LEAVES—A BEAUTY ELIXIR THAT HYDRATES THE SKIN AND LIFTS THE MOOD

Spa treatments are a terrific way to relax and treat yourself. I love going to spas. When I travel and have a tight, busy schedule, I always try to finish my day with a facial, pedicure, and massage (hot/cold stone massage is superrelaxing).

After a couple of hours at the spa, I feel I'm in Heaven. My mind and body are totally relaxed and I'm ready to fall asleep. Those nights, I don't need to count a single sheep!

Learn to do at-home spa treatments as an alternative to the real spa experience, which can require money and time that you don't have. I perform my home spa regimen every morning: I drop bath salts into warm running water and relax in the bathtub for 10 to 15 minutes. I use body products that uplift me, such as lemongrass and lavender body scrubs. The scents wake me up, make me feel great, and put me in a good mood for the rest of the day. I also do a home facial in the bathtub, under the running water, including cleansing and exfoliation. I follow with a hydrating mask that I leave on my face for 15 minutes after bathing.

Donna Shoemaker, *Spa director, Serenitè Spa, Sedona, Arizona. The Spa to L'Auberge de Sedona and Amara Hotel.*

## HERE'S HOW TO PAMPER YOURSELF WITH AN AT-HOME SPA.

### Preparation

1. The spa experience appeals to all five senses: hearing, smell, taste, sight, and touch.

2. Create a heavenly atmosphere: pick out your favorite colored pillows, towels, blankets, candles, and flowers, and put petals into the bathtub or foot soak.

3. Scents can trigger memories and take you to another time and place. Use candles, oils, and/or incense, or you can simmer your favorite spices on the stove to fill your home with a natural aroma. Cinnamon, clove, and nutmeg are great to add comfort and warm up on a cold day. Mint provides a cleansing, cooling feeling on a hot day.

4. You can create an Asian, tropical, or modern feel in your home spa: maybe all you need is some bamboo shoots or tropical flowers in your bathroom. A Buddha statue and a burning candle are very relaxing and give the feel of an Asian-style spa.

5. Playing music can deeply move you to feel what is right for you. After you set the tone for your home spa, try a little stretching. A round of the Sun Salutation, a great yoga move, can awaken the senses and relieve stress and muscle tension. Breathe. Take a few easy, deep breaths, and then, throughout your relaxing spa, be aware of your breathing. If you find your thoughts becoming stressful or worrisome, refocus on your breathing. Keep your attention focused on the experience of your senses, and let everything else go.

6. Before you go shopping, check your drawers and cabinets for products and samples you've forgotten about. Much of what you need can be found in your kitchen: sea salt, herbs, olive oil, coffee, honey, and eggs.

    a. A colorful fruit or vegetable salad is a great choice for your home spa lunch. Or maybe you prefer a dark chocolate mousse. Have the food ready before the home spa starts, because you don't want to spend your precious time chopping vegetables or peeling oranges.

    b. Remember to drink pure water. You may want to enhance the water with lemons, limes, cucumbers, ginger, and/or mint, or choose herbal noncaffeinated teas such as licorice, mint, ginger, or green tea. Staying hydrated will help you feel and look your absolute best! Keep a bottle of water with you at all times.

7. If you don't have a hot tub or sauna, don't fret. Any bathroom, bedroom, or living room can be transformed into an oasis of luxury with a little imagination.

8. Get a babysitter for your kids or pets (maybe for your husband as well . . . ).

9. Get into your most comfortable clothes for your spa. A soft robe, sweats, an extra-large T-shirt—whatever makes you feel relaxed.

Don't forget your socks or slippers, and maybe a ribbon or a colorful wrap for your hair.

**10.** Unplug the phone, lock the doors, and, whatever you do, don't get on the scale.

## Treatments

**1.** Dry brush to remove dry skin and stimulate blood flow.

**2.** Bathe or shower (not too hot). Afterward, polish your skin with a loofah or body scrub. If you don't have these items, you can use sea salt or kosher salt mixed with oil. Use green organic ground coffee mixed into olive oil and a dash of your favorite essential oil or herb for scent. I like the salt combination for the shower or tub to enhance your soak.

**3.** Coffee is better for the shower. To exfoliate the skin, use organic ground coffee mixed with olive oil. Caffeine has antioxidant properties for the skin, but soaking in it isn't recommended, as you will absorb the caffeine and probably won't be able to rest afterward. Also, if you have sensitive skin or you have shaved/waxed, salt can sting.

**4.** Other options for the tub include bath salts, Epsom salt, essential oils, flower petals, and bubbles, if you are in the mood for a bubble bath.

**5.** If you choose the tub or if you have a steam room or sauna, have some cool towels, perhaps wrapped in ice with cucumbers, ready to apply to the back of your neck to keep your temperature balanced. Overheating can cause a headache and ruin the moment.

**6.** Pat yourself dry and follow with massage oil, moisturizer, or maybe some Tiger Balm if you have sore muscles. Focus on the dry areas, such as heels, knees, and elbows.

**7.** For the face, start with a gentle cleansing with warm water and follow with exfoliation. A gentle massage with a washcloth can also be effective. Bring a pot filled with an inch of water to a boil. Remove and set on a stable surface so you can sit with your clean face over the steam. Drape a towel over your head to hold the steam in. This will bring moisture to the skin and open and clear your pores.

**8.** Adding essential oils can enhance your steam treatment. Chamomile

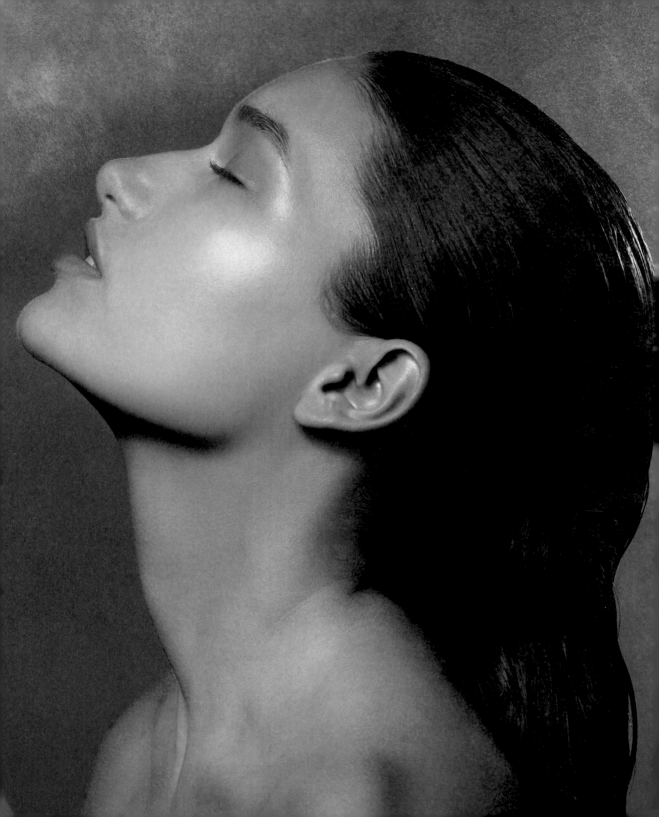

is soothing, whereas peppermint with tea tree oil will clear the sinuses. Follow the steam treatment with your favorite mask. Clay masks are good to clear clogged pores, but for combination skin, use them only in your T-zone and apply a moisturizing mask to the rest of the face. Egg white makes a good tightening mask, whereas egg yolks with honey make a better moisturizing mask. Lie down for 15 to 20 minutes, close your eyes, and really relax.

9.   After rinsing off the mask, use a toner followed with a serum and your skin type's moisturizer and eye cream.

10.   Try a deep-conditioning treatment and a deep-conditioning hair mask. You can also hit your own kitchen for olive oil, mayo, or avocado! Try them as a scalp/hair treatment with massage. Put a plastic cap on your head and add a towel wrap to keep the heat in. Shampoo the treatment out. Your hair may initially be a bit flat, but another shampoo will make it look shiny and healthy again.

11.   Healthy hair is happy hair and a sign of good overall health. If you are heavy-handed with finishing products, an occasional clarifying shampoo is a good treatment. If you have colored hair, make sure it's color-safe.

12.   Rest is an important element. White, clean sheets are pure luxury right after the treatments. If you can't afford sheets with a high thread count, wash yours with unscented fabric softener, with a few drops of essential oil added. I like to treat the edges of sheets and pillowcases with my favorite essential oils. Lavender is lovely for clearing your mind and relaxing. Sleep is our best defense against aging. It's our rejuvenation time.

13.   Manicures and pedicures can also be included in your home spa treatment (see chapter 6, "Manicures and Pedicures").

## SHORT LIST OF TREATMENTS

Be creative in mixing and matching the treatments in your home spa.

Dry brush your body, add oil to your hair, and then slip into the bath.
Exfoliate your face and apply a mask. Enjoy a little spa cuisine while soaking.

Massage a sea salt and oil mixture on your entire body, paying attention to your feet and other rough, dry areas (a body scrub/exfoliating cream will also do the same job). Rinse off the mask and hair oil in the tub, towel dry, tone and moisturize the face and body, wrap up in something comfy including a hat or head wrap to stay warm, push back your cuticles, shape and buff your nails, put on white cotton gloves, and retire for the evening. In the morning I shampoo and shower before applying sunscreen to face the fabulous new day!

# Hisako Minervini, Esthetician

### EYE-AREA TREATMENTS

Use an eye-area mask along with the face mask. This will soften and relax the sensitive, thin skin around the eyes. Follow with an eye-area cream or gel. The eye-area skin will look firmer and more relaxed and youthful.

An eye-area mask is a good product to use, especially in the winter, when the skin around the eyes tends to be dry. Apply a thicker layer of the product by tapping the cream with your ring finger from the outside corner inward, toward your nose. On the eyelid, do the reverse, from the nose outward. Make a circle like a doughnut, but once again, the direction is very important, because the eye muscle is like a ring and the application of the cream must follow the direction of the eye muscle. You don't want to go against it.

Use very gentle pressure, as mentioned earlier, because the skin around the eye area is very thin and sensitive. Do not move the skin! Don't think you must massage the eye cream into the skin. Your under-eye skin is not supposed to move. If you move the skin with too much pressure, you will end up with wrinkles. Leave the mask on for 10 to 15 minutes, and then press tissue on the skin to absorb the excess cream.

The other option is eye-area pads, which are also great for traveling. They hydrate the skin very well.

*Start using eye cream—the sooner the better. Around twenty years of age is a good time to start using eye-area treatments.*

*To remove dark circles on mature skin, you want to get more hydration and also soften the fine lines. For young and oily skin, use an oil-free, light-textured liquid or gel base.*

### How to Apply Eye-Area Cream Correctly
*Use your ring finger, because you can control the application better and it's weak enough not to give too much pressure.*

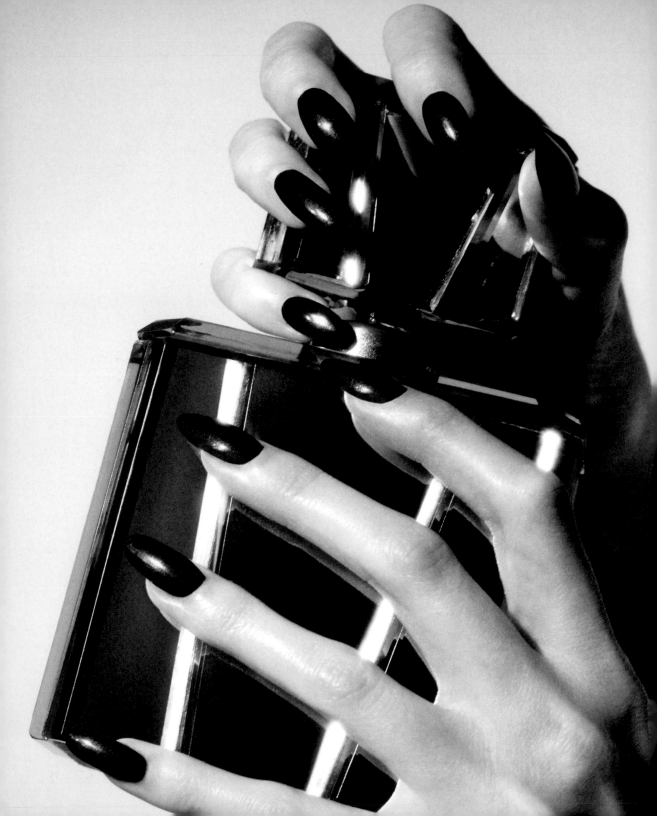

# 6 MANICURES AND PEDICURES

**It's easy and relaxing to have your mani-pedicure done by a professional, so you can sit back and read the latest gossip magazines or just relax. But you can also do it yourself.**

**Beth Fricke,** *celebrity manicurist at OPI, Los Angeles*

Your hands and feet are used all day, every day, and need to be loved and cared for like all other parts of the body. When your hands and feet look good, they contribute a part of your fabulous total look.

Note: A good manicurist can help you determine the overall health of your nails and can refer you to a doctor if there are any problems.

## TOOLS OR EQUIPMENT NEEDED FOR A MANICURE/PEDICURE

**Nail clippers:** to trim nails to an even length
**Nail file:** to smooth and shape the nails (nonmetal, 180 grit or higher)
**Buffer:** to smooth the tops of the nails (220 grit or higher)
**Nail brush:** to brush and exfoliate cuticles
**Orangewood stick:** to clean under the nails and correct polish errors
**Foot file/pumice:** to smooth and remove dead skin from calluses
**Cuticle nippers:** to trim hangnails and dead skin (use as little as possible)
**Buffer:** to shine the nails for the look of clear polish

## PRODUCTS NEEDED FOR A MANICURE/PEDICURE

**Oil:** to moisturize/condition the cuticles and nails
**Lotion:** to moisturize hands and feet
(especially after foot file/pumice/scrub use)

ORANGEWOOD STICK >>>

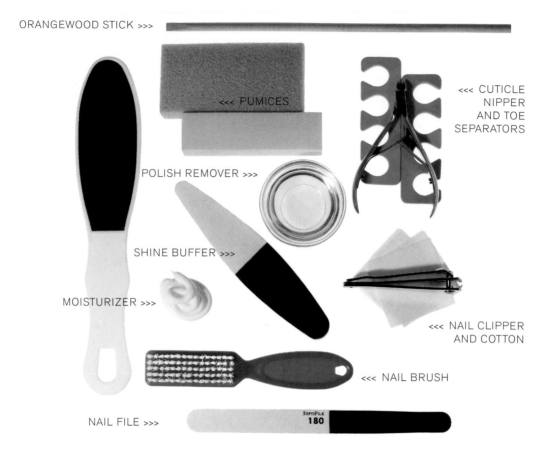

<<< PUMICES

<<< CUTICLE
NIPPER
AND TOE
SEPARATORS

POLISH REMOVER >>>

SHINE BUFFER >>>

MOISTURIZER >>>

<<< NAIL CLIPPER
AND COTTON

NAIL FILE >>>

SeptiFile
180

<<< NAIL BRUSH

**Polish remover:** to remove polish and prep the nails for polishing
**Base Coat:** to prime the nail for polish and to prevent polish staining
**Top Coat:** to even out and seal in the polish

Soak your hands or feet in water (or do the mani-pedicure after a shower or bath); brush and massage your cuticles with a nail brush. Trim your nails to an even length with a nail clipper. (If you wear polish, try to visualize the nails with polish—the nail bed length can vary.) File your nails to the desired shape, following the line of your nails (between the pink and white) for a natural look. Clean under the nails with the orangewood stick. Make sure there are no hidden points, and retrim any ruffles with your file. Buff the tops of the nails from the cuticle to the free edge with your buffer to make them smooth and create a better surface for polish or buffing. If you must use nippers, now is the time. Remember to trim only skin that is standing up or hanging loose; the rest needs to be there to protect your nail and hold it on.

You may also use a wet foot file or pumice on damp feet—just on the rough spots! You are only removing dead skin, not the calluses, which need to be there to protect your feet from the weight of your body. You just want them to be smooth! Once your feet are smooth, don't forget to apply lotion (the replacement for the skin you just removed).

### How often do nails need to be maintained?

Most natural and artificial nails should be attended to by a professional every couple of weeks. You may need to do some maintenance of your own once or twice a week, but it should just be touch-up filing, moisturizing, and possibly applying top coat.

### How long should polish last?

We manicurists should be able to guarantee fingernails for a couple of days, toes for a few weeks, but if a mani-pedicure is done correctly, fingernails should last a week and toes six weeks.

The nails should be buffed with your soft buffer and wiped with acetone, getting in to the sides and across the tips of the nail. Use a good base coat (such as Sticky by Creative Nail Design), two thin coats of fresh polish, and a good, solid top coat (such as Seche Vite). Bottles of nail polish can last for years as long as the bottle tops are cleaned off so no air can get in and they are stored in a cool, dry place.

### Are there any diseases or restrictions related to nail care services?

Diabetes patients require more care, as they are more prone to infection. Ingrown nails require special care and cannot be cut into! Allergies I see are usually not from polish but from other things, such as allergies to fragrances or mold from improper nail prep before the application of extensions. I also see fungus resulting from too-intense cleaning products or, even worse, unclean tools or tubs.

### What can I do about stinky feet?

Wash the ankles, the feet, and between the toes with a washcloth or shower scrunchie during every shower or bath.

### I'm on vacation, and my nails look terrible. What can I do?

The quick fix is to file your nails as needed, apply another top coat (don't forget to seal in the tips), and smother the nails with cuticle oil. Oil fixes a lot and will make the nails look supple.

### What is the difference between a French manicure and a regular manicure?

The only difference is the polish. A regular manicure should include either buff or single polish. In a French manicure, white polish is applied to the tip and a soft pink is laid over the top. If your manicurist can do it freehand, you have other color choices as well—for example, a red nail with a black tip or a white pearl nail with a navy tip.

### What are the best nail polish color choices for fair/medium/dark skin tones?

All colors are open to everyone. Which color is chosen really depends on one's personal style. Sometimes a person who normally wears light pinks wants to have electric blue nails, because she's going to a party and will be wearing a denim dress and open-toed high heels. Nail color is like an accessory: go with your moods and styles.

> **Fair skin:** Light pink/pastel sheer colors, true reds, and darker colors in mauves, burgundies, and purples work well.
> **Medium skin:** Sheer pinks and corals, cool-tone deep reds, and browns work well.
> **Dark skin:** Sheers with white or peach, jewel tones, bright fuchsia, and reds work extremely well. For a darker nail color, I usually go with ruby, wine, or brown.

### What are some options for sporty/active people?

Keep your nails short. Extensions will just be broken during activity, further damaging the nails, so why bother? Many women are active these days, and short nails are the cool thing.

### What are the options for extensions?

If you want really long ones, tips with acrylic overlays are the best. For just a little length, I love a good freehand acrylic (using a form). I know that power drills have gained popularity in the last few years, and most people use them now, but as far as I am concerned there is never a reason to use a power tool on your body or your nails. Drills are the reason acrylics now get a bad rap, when they can actually be a healthy, beautiful thing, if done correctly.

If you are looking for something less rigid, a good choice is gel. For good support for your own nails and extensions with a tip, the gels can be really nice. They're like a thick polish that is cured under a light. They now even come in colors for a more durable polished look!

### What about the nails one can buy at the grocery store or drugstore?

They can be used. They tend not to look natural, but if you can make them work, go, girl! The only thing is that artificial nails are a lot about the nail prep, and that can go wrong. One of my best clients had those nails—she had turned green underneath!

### It's so hard to paint one's own nails . . . any tricks?

Do not go all the way to the edge of the cuticle, especially at the base of the nail. Bring the touch of the brush to the middle of the nail, and then spread it from there.

Use two thin coats of polish—it will dry much faster than one thick one—although sometimes I do use only one coat on the nails if it's a sheer polish. Use your pinky finger to balance your hand for more control. And keep your orangewood stick handy; if you wipe off a mistake as soon as you make it, you won't have to go over it later with remover. And don't forget to run the brush over the tip of the nail on the first coat of polish to help seal the polish and make it look nicer.

### Why does one need a base or top coat?

A good base coat is thin and sticky. It acts as a primer for the polish, helping it adhere to the nail and preventing staining of the nails by darker polish. A good top coat will even out the polish and seal it in. The top coat needs to be thick and protective but fast-drying.

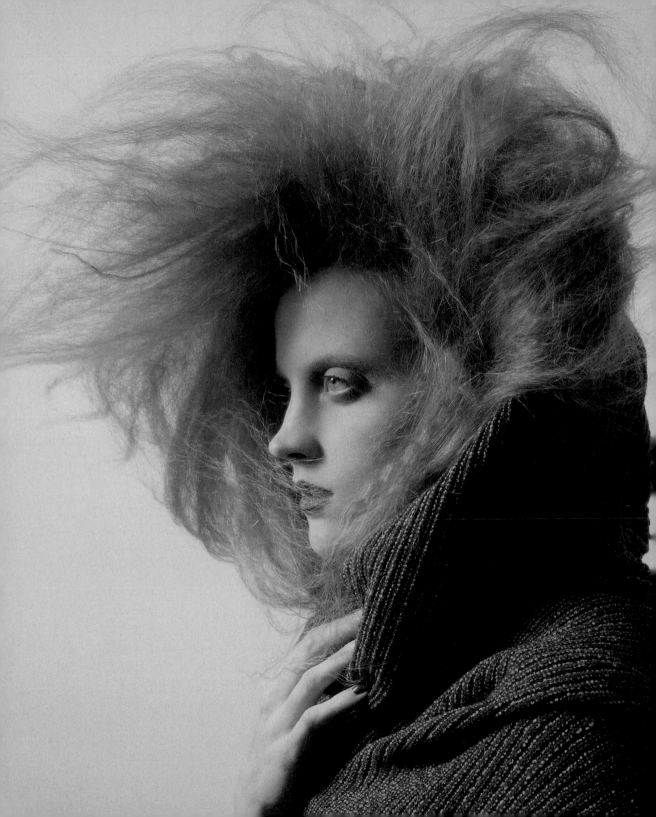

# 7 HAIR

PHOTO: KURT ISWARIENKO/MODEL: LINDSAY @ PHOTOGENICS/HAIR: LOUISE MOON/NAILS: BETH FRICKE/STYLING: HEIDI MEEK

**I have been lucky to work with some of the leading hairstylists in the world. Whether creating an elegant French '60s updo or a simple bohemian hairstyle, they always make the hair look simply amazing.**

One of the stylists is the Malaysian-born hair guru Kevin Woon, whose beautiful hairstyles have been seen in many fashion and beauty magazines. He is also well known for his excellent haircutting techniques. When he is not creating hairdos on the set, he is working on his clients at his SoHo salon in New York City.

**Kevin Woon,** *Woon Salon, New York City*

**Michael Anthony,** *master colorist, Woon Salon*

The first step in discerning which hairstyle suits a particular client who steps into our salon for the first time is conversation. I ask questions about her lifestyle: what her profession is, if she travels a lot, if she goes to a gym or does other sports and activities. Also, I ask if she has time to do her own hair in the morning. Most women don't. I also take into consideration the texture, length, and thickness of her hair. Hair texture helps me decide what kind of cut and shape I should do and create, how many layers it can handle to keep the shape and length. I like to create a hairstyle that brings out the best in a person, one she can maintain until the next haircut. In short, I look for the unique characteristics we all have and create a hairstyle that shows individuality.

## FULLER IS BETTER
Coloring can give a 3-D effect that makes the hair look fuller, playing with the depth of the tone and the contrast. If your hair is superthin, supplements such as vitamin

B6 and B12, seaweed, and a healthy diet help. However, I would suggest seeking professional help from a nutritionist or doctor for the best advice on nutrition.

*Does it make a difference if I buy my shampoos, conditioners, and styling products at a salon or at a drugstore?*

It can. When you purchase any kind of hair product from a hair salon, the product is recommended to you by your stylist, who knows exactly what your hair needs. The stylist knows this because she or he has tried it and therefore can help you find specific products for your hair type and needs. Also, purchasing hair products from a salon guarantees you an authentic product.

## SHAMPOO

**Dry shampoo** was developed for situations in which people cannot wash their hair with liquid shampoo and water. Dry shampoo usually comes in a spray. Its powderlike consistency attaches itself to the grease and dirt in your hair so you can brush the dirt away. It also deodorizes. This is just a quick fix; eventually the person must use liquid shampoo and water. At photo shoots dry shampoo is kept handy in case the hair needs a little bit more body; using it can really fluff the hair!

**Blue shampoo:** On the color wheel, blue is almost opposite yellow. We suggest that a client use this shampoo if she is experiencing yellowing of her hair color, or to neutralize or balance the color. This is most apparent on blondes, especially on highlighted or bleached-blonde hair. This may be caused by the water they wash their hair with, especially if their plumbing is old and there is rust in the water, or they may secrete an excess of keratin, the waxy secretion, Mother Nature's conditioner, that when combined with sweat makes hair greasy. The color of keratin is yellow.

*What can I do to combat hair loss?*

Start by seeing trichologist (hair doctor). Hair transplants have improved a lot, and it's worth looking into that option, although it's quite expensive.

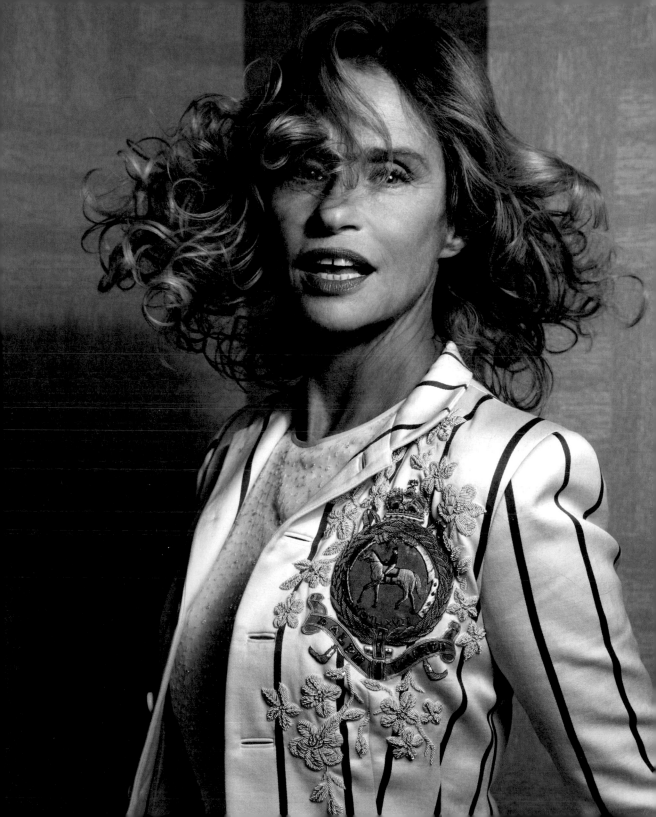

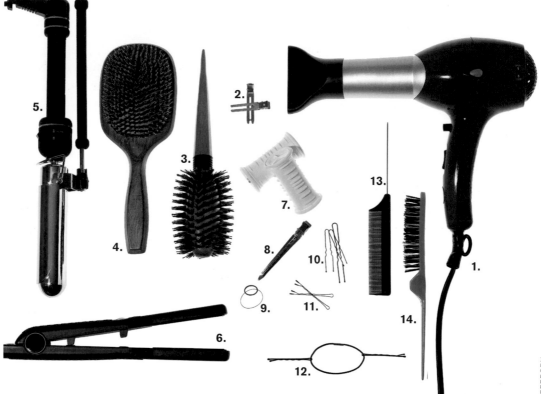

1. IONIC BLOW DRYER 2. HAIR CLIPS FOR PIN CURLS 3. ROUND BRUSH FOR BLOW DRYING 4. FLAT BRUSH FOR BLOW DRYING THE HAIR STRAIGHT, BRUSHING THE HAIR, AND OPENING CURLS 5. CURLING IRON 6. FLATIRON 7. HOT ROLLERS 8. LARGE SECTIONING CLIP FOR SEPARATING THE HAIR WHILE WORKING WITH HOT TOOLS 9. SMALL RUBBER BANDS 10. ANGEL-WING PINS 11. BOBBY PINS 12. ONE RUBBER BAND WITH A BOBBY PIN ON EACH END IS THE SECRET TO A LONG-LASTING PONYTAIL 13. TEASING COMB WITH A METAL SPIKE HANDLE THAT YOU CAN USE FOR SEPARATING THE HAIR (GOOD ALSO FOR CREATING SIDE AND MIDDLE PARTINGS) 14. SMALL HAIRBRUSH FOR OPENING THE CURLS, BRUSHING THROUGH THE CURLS

PHOTO: KIINO VILLAND/PROP STYLIST: MATHILDA CHRISTOFFERSEN

*How much does hair grow in a month?*

About ¼ inch.

*Can Asian hair be permed?*

Permed hair is very popular in the Asian community. However, certain precautions should be taken beforehand. Your hairstylist should examine your hair and scalp carefully to determine whether you are a good candidate for a perm.

## HOME TRICKS

When you step out of a salon, your hair looks amazing—but not necessarily after the first wash, when you have no idea how to style it. Your hairstylist should always show you how to do your hair by demonstrating some basic techniques. I sometimes even let my clients blow-dry their own hair while I watch and guide them.

### THE FAST WAY TO BLOW-DRY HAIR AT HOME

Predry your hair to around 80 percent dry, and then use a round brush if you want some volume and wave or a Mason Pearson brush for a straighter style.

*How can I keep a rubber band from slipping off a ponytail?*

Get a rubber band that looks like a bungee cord with a hook on each end. Hook each end on the base of the ponytail, and then wrap the rubber band around until you feel it's tight enough. Finally, attach the other hook on the base. You can also use a regular rubber band, attach a bobby pin on each end, and follow the instructions above.

## BANGS

*Want fashionable Chrissie Hynde–style bangs, but have a strong cowlick?*

Stylists should avoid cutting bangs unless the person is willing to train them; otherwise they won't work. Depending on the direction of the cowlick, sometimes changing the parting of the hair can solve the problem. However, for a stubborn bang, it's best to comb the hair down or in the direction of your part right after shampooing. Blow-dry the bang in the direction of your part.

## BIGGEST HAIR CRIMES

Too many layers

Overprocessing

Too trendy

### *How important is the collaboration between the hairstylist and the colorist?*

The chemistry and vision of the two must be complementary for the best effect. The cut creates shape and movement; color provides dimension.

### *What is the difference between semipermanent color and permanent color?*

The difference is the size of the color molecule and how it enters the hair shaft. Semipermanent color molecules are larger in size than permanent and usually need heat to open the hair in order to allow the molecule to enter because there is no ammonia release from a developer.

### *How do I know which hair color will suit me?*

Hair color is picked for many different reasons. The number one reason is to cover gray hair. There is actually no such thing as gray hair. Individual hairs are white, not gray; it's the background that makes them appear gray.

Colorists call this the client's base color. The base color is picked to suit the skin color and age of the client. For dimension on a base color, colorists do lowlights and highlights, usually in the same tonal family as the base color, for natural highs and lows that will give dimension to the color.

### *Why is it so important to use color shampoo and conditioner instead of regular ones?*

Some shampoos and conditioners are specifically made for color-treated hair. They are formulated with gentler detergents that are more moisturizing, and they usually contain a sunscreen. Some shampoos and conditioners for color-treated hair include small amounts of color. This helps maintain the color for longer periods of time, especially for people who spend a lot of time in the sun.

### How often should I see my colorist?

I recommend every four to six weeks for a touch-up. That's about how long it takes the original color to show through. Roots that have grown out for four to six weeks are usually around ½ inch long. Highlight and lowlight touch-ups, if done right, can last as long as three or four months.

### Can salt water and sun damage highlighted hair?

Highlights are usually put in by a discoloration process using either bleach or a high lift color, and we also carefully place tone into the highlights to balance the highlights with the base color. Without sunscreen protection, the sun will further bleach the hair and lift out the tone the colorist created. Salt water has a drying effect over time if the hair is not well washed and conditioned. Dry hair makes your color look faded and old.

### Why doesn't red color stay in hair well?

Red is the hardest color to lift out of the hair, and the hardest color to keep. The reason is the weight of the color molecule: the darker the color, the heavier the weight of the color molecule. Dark brown fades as well, but the weight of the color molecule is heavier, and thus it fades more slowly. Reds are lighter and thus fade quickly; blonde is the lightest and fades just as fast, but it doesn't have the same intensity as red so it's not as noticeable. When red is freshly done, it's the most intense color. Reds are my personal favorites and the colors I enjoy doing the most.

The way to keep your red color longer is to get frequent touch-ups and use a shampoo and conditioner for color-treated hair. Stay out of direct sun, and every once in a while get a color glaze. Color glazes are translucent colors that help seal color in and condition the hair. I love the shine and depth of color they bring to the hair.

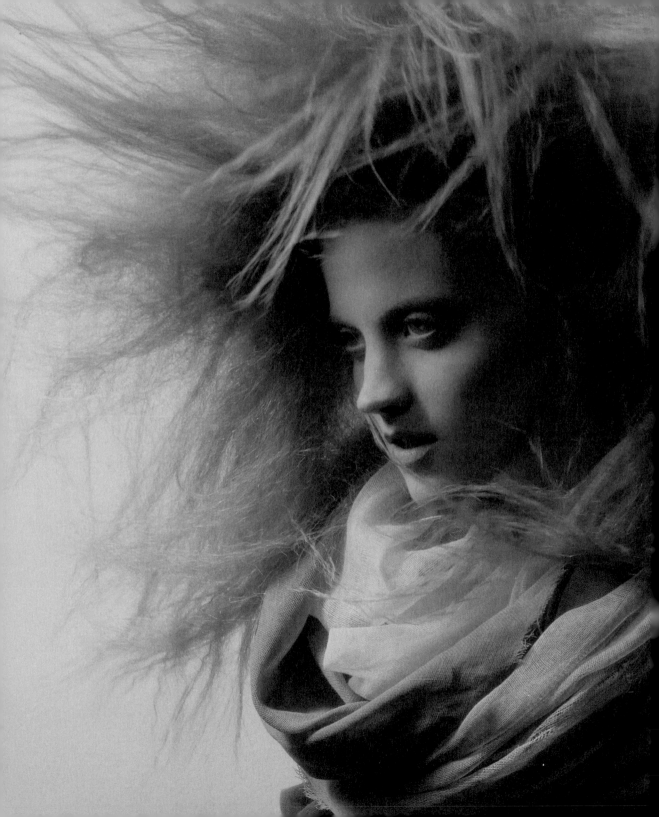

# HAIR EXTENSIONS AND WIGS

**LOUISE MOON,** *hairstylist and extension specialist at Sally Herschberger Salon, LA*

Hair extensions are a serious option for getting longer, thicker hair with very natural-looking results. Extensions were used by the Egyptians as early as 3400 B.C. Wigs and extensions were made of human hair or even sheep's wool. During the mid–eighteenth century, hairstyles were massive, requiring added-on human hair. Wigs, hairpieces, and extensions made a comeback again in the twentieth century thanks to the silent movie queen Mary "America's Sweetheart" Pickford, who made long ringlets very fashionable for young ladies in the 1920s. Hairpieces and extensions were used through every decade, but 1960s hairstyles really boosted extensions into fashion: big hairpieces and extensions were placed under and on top of the hair to get fuller, thicker, and more massive hairstyles. Remember Jane Fonda in *Barbarella,* and the hairpieces and extensions she wore! In the 1980s, Antenna Salon in London created the new extension culture for pop stars such as Bananarama, Boy George, and Marilyn. And the rest of the world followed: Cyndi Lauper and Madonna.

The types of attachments vary, depending on your budget, hair quality, reason for adding hair, and comfort. There are different textures, colors, densities, qualities, and attachments. There are individual bonds, which can be applied anywhere on the head to add volume, length, or color. They are very comfortable and can be moved easily to put the hair up or back. The attachment can be the size of half a baby's fingernail, or even finer. There are pretipped bond attachments and plastic and metal bead attachments for braiding your own hair into the extension hair. Another option is a weft. This is a long roll of hair, cut to whatever width you need. This is a less costly option that can add a lot of hair very quickly. There are wefts that you sew into your braided "track" hair. There are also wefts that you can clip into your hair to wear for the day and wefts that you use a special tape to attach the hair, which lasts a while.

### Are there any reasons extensions can't be used?
If you are losing hair for whatever reason, adding extensions will only aggravate

the loss. If your hair is very fine, it may not have the strength to hold the weight of the attached hair or will not be able to conceal the attachment. Brittle hair is a problem as well.

### What is the minimum length for hair to take extensions?
You need at least 3½ to 4 inches of hair to conceal the attachment.

### How long do extensions last, and how often should I see a stylist to treat my roots?
It depends on what type of extensions you have and how fast your hair grows. Do *not* go longer than the stylist tells you, to avoid breakage of your own hair. Wefts can last anywhere from one to two months maximum. Individual pretips can last three to five months, depending on how thick the bond is.

### Can extensions be dyed or highlighted?
Yes, but you really need to be aware of the quality of the hair and how well it will respond to the color.

### How about using a curling iron or blow-drying?
You can; just be careful not to put heat on the attachment base if it is a bond attachment, and also pay attention to how much tension you are putting on the hair while blow-drying.

### How about sleeping with extensions; don't they get messy?
Well, it can be a "nightmare" if you go to bed with wet hair! *Never* do that. Long hair can be more of a problem than short. I suggest a scrunchie to pull your dry hair into a low ponytail, or you can plait your hair into two braids. Also, a satin pillowcase can help.

### What if my extensions fail? Are there any tricks to put them back by myself?
Ummm, no. You must see a professional.

### Is there any danger of the extensions damaging my own hair?

Yes, if they are not put in right. Too much tension, or uneven tension, or even too-heavy hair, can cause breakage. Clients should be fully educated on how to care for their extensions. Also, leaving extensions in the hair too long can be harmful. You shed hair every day, 100 to 200 hairs a day! The more shedding you do, the less hair is holding the attached hair. Too much tension is put on the remaining hair, and then breakage can occur. When the hairdresser says to come back in three months—do so! Also, if you do not brush and separate your hair from the root, the hair shed at the base of the attachment will start to knot. This will cause breakage, and this is probably the problem most people face. Brushing your hair with a boar-bristle brush can help.

### How much do extensions cost?

It depends on the stylist's time, what type of extension it is, and the hair quality, density, color, texture, and, of course, length.

## HOLLYWOOD HAIR

**ROBERTO RAMOS,** *Estilo Salon, Los Angeles*

Braids—little or thick French or ordinary braids—are being used in every way possible. Hollywood remains an influence on trends and styles. The hairstyles of stars are redone exactly or used as inspiration. Hair today is healthy and lush. It isn't greasy or filled with products. Hair is also moving toward a fuller look with more body, away from the flat-on-the-head and flatironed-to-death look.

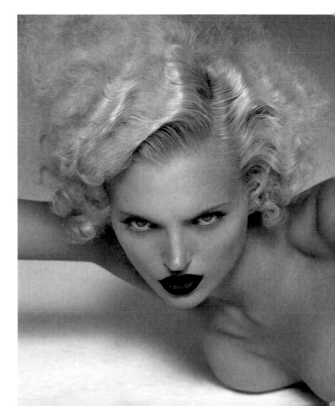

# THREE POPULAR LOOKS ON THE RED CARPET THESE DAYS

### Straight

Use spray leave-in conditioner; this will help straighten and protect the hair. Blow-dry with a big round boar-bristle hairbrush to smooth the hair and help it straighten. If you want, you can use a ceramic flatiron to achieve a silky-straight look.

### Wavy

Use the leave-in conditioner while the hair is wet, for protection. Then use a special volumizer product (which I used to achieve Jessica Alba's look) at the roots and midshaft to get fullness and texture. Then blow-dry while scrunching the hair with or without a diffuser. This will help give you the body and texture you want.

Then use a ceramic curling iron to start waving the hair. A smaller iron gives more curl; a bigger iron gives wave. I used a 1-inch barrel on Jessica to get her waves. Remember always to curl the hair in the opposite direction so that the curls or waves will stay separate.

### Updo

To achieve an updo, you don't always need clean hair. It actually works better on one-day-"old" hair. There are different ways to create an updo, but what is needed is the volume that can be achieved by teasing, curling, or hot roller setting the hair and, definitely, using a volumizer. From there on, it will be a personal choice how you want to create the updo: twists, braids, and French braids can all be incorporated into an updo. I use a special texturizing cream for texturizing and smoothing the hair. Use hairpins (angel hairpins are the best, along with bobby pins) to hold the updo. Finish the updo by spraying it with a styling spray.

### *My hair gets oily very fast. What can I do?*

Use a dry shampoo to help keep the oil under control. Also, use a shampoo and conditioner for oily hair. Use the conditioner on the ends only and/or dilute the conditioner with water; this will help keep your hair from getting oily too soon.

## How can I straighten black, naturally curly hair?

There are many ways to do this. You can blow-dry and/or flatiron the hair. There are also various chemical hair straighteners available.

## What is the most damaging procedure for the hair?

Chemical straightening and bleaching the hair platinum. These two procedures really deplete nutrients from the hair. It's very important to get the hair into shape by using conditioners and deep-moisturizing masks before and after these treatments. Note: Always tell your stylist about any previous colors, highlights, and other chemical treatments, even if the treatment was applied a while ago. If not, your hair could become very damaged.

## The Effect of Humidity on Your Hairstyle

If you live in a place that is very humid and you want to keep your naturally wavy hair straight, chemical hair straighteners can change your life! They will cut down your blow-dry time. A flatiron used with some silicone drops will help keep the hair straight if you prefer not to take the chemical route.

## The Best Uplifting Hair Tricks for 50+ Women

Go a bit lighter, especially around the face, which always helps brighten the face and give a more youthful look. Try to stay away from too-dark or harsh colors. Also stay away from too-short or too-long hairstyles.

Try not to crowd your face with a lot of hair, as if you were hiding it. It will only emphasize your age. I suggest light, airy, off-the-face hairstyles because they give you a freer, more confident look.

Use a great shampoo and conditioner as well as a deep conditioner once a week. This will keep your hair in great shape, and supershiny.

# 8 FACE

The shape of our face is defined by our individual bone structure. Beautiful faces come in every shape.

Understanding your facial shape and bone structure will help you enhance your own individual beauty. It has been said that the oval face shape is the easiest to make up and the classiest, but I don't believe in such categorizing. There is no easy or difficult face shape. All are different, and all are beautiful. Most of us have a combination of face shapes, such as oval on the top, round on the bottom.

Facial shapes are important in makeup only when applying blush: for most people, it works best on the apples of the cheeks, or sometimes just under the cheeks, or in the hollow of the cheeks to give a contour (for round and square face shapes). But be light-handed in all cases.

Facial shapes are more important in finding a hairstyle. The right cut can shorten a long face, make a round face look less so, or diminish the prominence of the wide forehead in a heart-shaped face.

## FAMOUS FACIAL SHAPES

1. Round face: Isabella Rossellini
2. Long face: Sarah Jessica Parker
3. Heart-shaped face: Reese Witherspoon
4. Square face: Demi Moore
5. Oval face: Jessica Alba

Hair color can have an impact too. Sometimes highlights or a darker color, along with the proper haircut, enhance a facial shape.

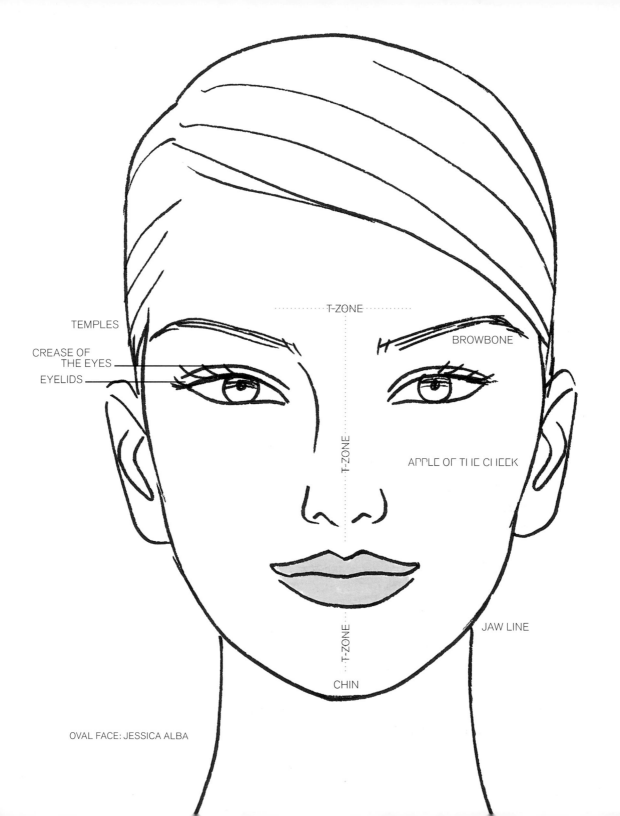

TEMPLES

CREASE OF
THE EYES

EYELIDS

T-ZONE

BROWBONE

T-ZONE

APPLE OF THE CHEEK

JAW LINE

T-ZONE

CHIN

OVAL FACE: JESSICA ALBA

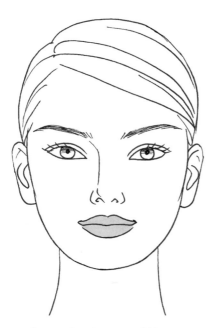

ROUND FACE: ISABELLA ROSSELLINI

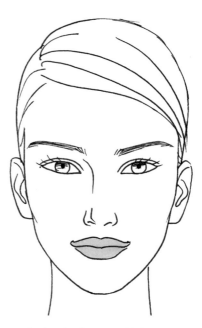

LONG FACE: SARAH JESSICA PARKER

## SOME IDEAS FOR STYLES

### Round Face

Keep the hair flat on the sides; round shapes make your face look even rounder. Avoid short bobs and curly, short hairstyles: they also make your face look rounder, and elongating your look is what you want to do.

### Long Face

Short bobs that cut the length of the face are great. Long bangs à la Chrissie Hynde flatter long face shapes as well. Avoid too-long and flat hair, though; it will drag you down. Pass on the teased big '80s Vogue hairdo, because it will stretch your face too much. Wavy or curly hair looks good because it gives width.

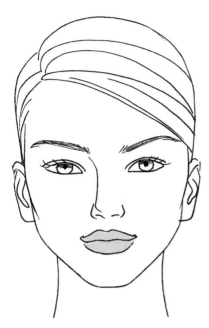

HEART-SHAPED FACE: REESE WITHERSPOON

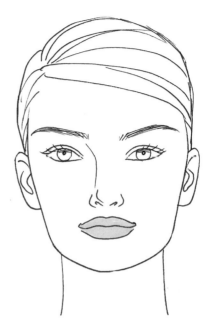

SQUARE FACE: DEMI MOORE

### Heart-shaped Face

Sideswept bangs look good for this facial shape, which has a wide forehead; avoid short hair, tight ponytails, short bangs, and short layers. Long hair and wavy long layers look the best.

### Square Face

Needs softer hairstyles, face-framing layers, wispy bangs, and fluffy curls. Avoid chin-length cuts, short Louise Brooks bobs, and one-length hairstyles.

### Oval Face

Any hairstyle looks fine: short, long, wavy, straight, bangs, sideswept, long bobs, short bobs.

# 9 TOOLS

The right tools will give you better results and make the application of makeup easier. We professionals can do our job using just our fingers and Q-tips (if we really have to), but it's important for you to have the right tools. I show the most important ones here. They are also my personal favorite tools. I use them regularly. You need brushes that are made of real hair (usually squirrel, pony, goat, weasel, sable, or kolinsky hair), as well as synthetic brushes (nylon or taklon).

*What makes a makeup brush good?*
A good brush for eye shadow, blush, powder, and lipstick is always made of real hair. Synthetics are for concealers, foundations, and lips. Synthetic brushes aren't good for powder-format makeup because the bristles can't hold the powders: they simply fall down, and your makeup will look like a big mess. You also can't blend, contour, or smudge well with synthetic brushes. Real-hair brushes hold powders well because their tips are uncut. The best powder-format brushes are handmade. They feel the softest on your skin and give you the best results.

*How should I take care of my brushes?*
Wash powders, waxes, and oils out of your brushes by using a regular bar soap and warm water. Wash them in the evening, and by morning they will be dry. Never lend your brushes to anyone because they are very personal items, just like lip gloss, lipstick, mascara or any other makeup or skin care product. I spray a professional brush cleaner on every brush every time before I use it. It sanitizes, deodorizes, and conditions, and also kills viruses and bacteria.

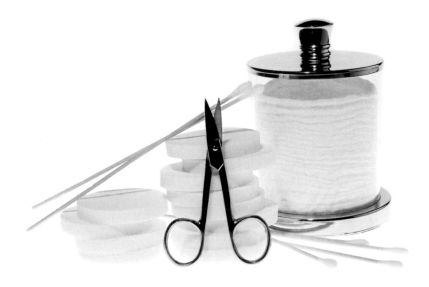

STILL LIFE: KIINO VILLAND/PROP STYLIST: MATHILDA CHRISTOFFERSEN

### How often should I wash my brushes?

It depends on how often you use them. If you use them every day, you should at least wipe them every day, and wash them one to three times a week. The best idea is to spray a brush cleaner on your brushes after every use and wipe them clean.

### How long will my brushes last?

As long as you take good care of them. Good brushes are expensive, especially those made of real hair, but they are an excellent investment because you will get much better results. I still use brushes I bought in 1988!

### Are Q-tips a good makeup tool?

Yes, for everything! For smoky eyes when you need to clean up the inner corners. You can also smudge eyeliner with a Q-tip, but be sure the cotton is pressed tight because otherwise there will be cotton fragments on your eyelids. Q-tips are excellent for cleaning off your eye makeup, especially liner that is "stuck" on the roots of your lashes. I also love the lip-makeup removal swabs. When you break the tip, the light-formula oil runs to the other side of the tip and it's ready to be used. It cleans off the lips superfast, and the oil leaves them moist. I also use the swabs on the eyes if I have made a mistake on the liner: I just break the tip and tap a clean Q-tip in the oil. That way I get just the smallest amount of oil, and it will remove the eyeliner from just the needed area. Q-tips and oil swabs (along with cleansing wipes) are great tools when you travel: you can clean your makeup fast and easily.

### Blotting paper

Blotting paper is used to reduce shine on your skin, eyelids, or lips. Just press the thin paper on the area, and it will absorb the oil and wax.

### Tweezers

Tweezerman is a brand of tweezers that are simply the best, including automatic tweezers. They automatically pull out those unwanted hairs by squeezing the side handles, and the slant tip tweezer reacts, removing the hair. Tweezerman also has free sharpening! Clean your tweezers after use by spraying them with brush cleaner and wiping them dry.

### Sponges

You need sponges to tap in foundation and give it the most natural look.
With a triangle sponge you can apply foundation in the corners of and under your eyes lightly better than by using a round one. But whichever you prefer will do. Use the sponge just once and then throw it away. Because most of the sponges are made of latex, they don't take warm water and soap very well. So make sure you have plenty of them in your makeup cabinet!

### Eyelash Curler

After every use, clean the rubber with a brush cleaner that contains alcohol. This removes all the bacteria. Some of them curl your lashes better and faster than others. My all-time favorite is the one from Shu Uemura. I also like the heated eyelash curlers, which are now very safe. The difference between the two is that with a traditional curler you apply mascara after you have curled your lashes, and with a heating curler you do the opposite. The corner curler works for all your lashes by curling them step by step in two to three sections from inside to outside corners. It's also a brilliant tool for curling any "leftover" lashes that don't fit into the regular-size curler. You must test them to find the one you like the best. And if you already have naturally beautifully waved lashes, you won't need these tools at all!

## Spatula/What does a spatula do?

It helps to get out the last bit of product, as well as helps to mix foundations and lipsticks.

**1.** POWDER PUFF **2.** TRIANGULAR NONLATEX MAKEUP SPONGE **3.** Q-TIPS **4.** LIP REMOVER SWABS THAT CONTAIN OIL; GOOD ALSO FOR REMOVING ANY MISTAKES ON EYE MAKEUP, SUCH AS MASCARA SPOTS AND UNEVEN LINERS **5.** BLOTTING PAPERS FOR TOUCH-UPS **6.** EYE AND LIP MAKEUP PENCIL SHARPENER **7.** SMALLER EYELASH CURLER THAT WORKS ON THE CORNERS THAT ARE HARD TO REACH WITH A REGULAR CURLER; THE CORNER CURLER WORKS AS WELL TO INTERCONNECT FAKE LASHES TO YOUR OWN LASHES **8.** SOAP FOR WASHING THE OILS AND WAXES FROM BRUSHES **9.** HEATED EYELASH CURLER **10.** FOUNDATION BRUSH (SYNTHETIC) **11.** CONCEALER BRUSH (SYNTHETIC) **12.** POWDER BRUSH **13.** BLUSH BRUSH **14.** EYE SHADOW BRUSH NO. 1 (FOR APPLYING) **15.** EYE SHADOW BRUSH NO. 2 (FOR BLENDING AND SMUDGING) **16.** EYE SHADOW BRUSH NO. 3 (FOR BLENDING THE CREASE) **17.** SMALL EYE BRUSH NO. 4 (FOR SMUDGING THE PENCIL LINER) **18.** SWIRL BRUSH FOR SEPARATING AND CLEANING THE LASHES RIGHT AFTER MASCARA APPLICATION **19.** EYELINER BRUSH **20.** LIP BRUSH **21.** SPATULA **22.** METALLIC EYELASH COMB **23.** CLASSIC EYELASH CURLER

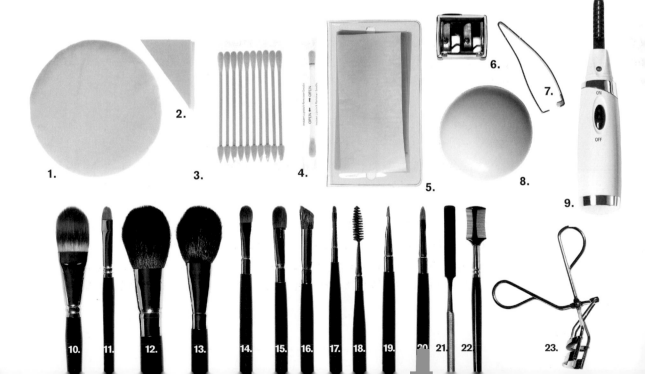

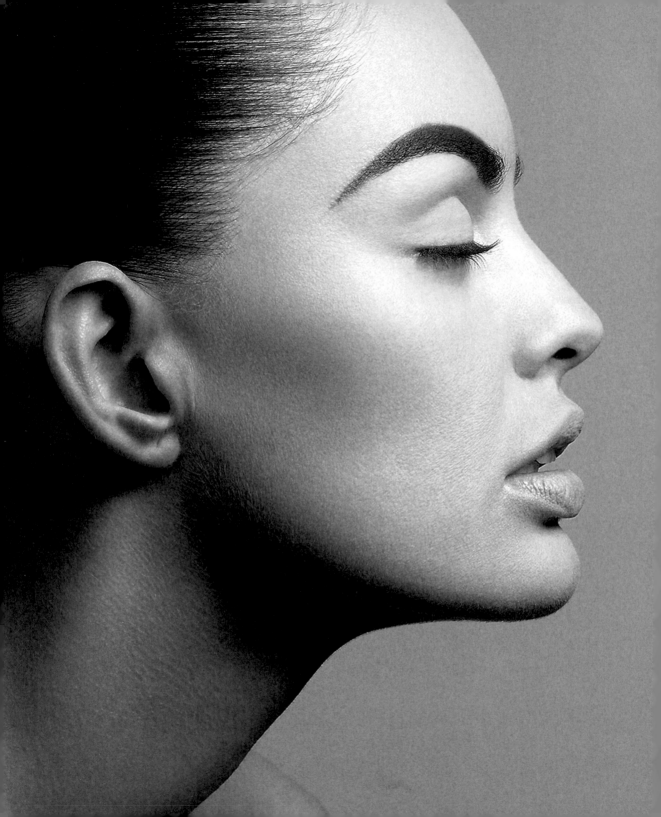

# 10 EYEBROWS

PHOTO: PASCAL DEMEESTER/MODEL: CAROLINA @ LA MODELS/HAIR: KEIKO HAMAGUCHI

**Eyebrows are probably the most important feature of your face. They frame your eyes, establishing a look and mood. Eyebrows can also give you an instant face-lift without surgery!**

Brow trends have changed over time. Brows have been shaved off, added to by using animal hair, and painted a rainbow of colors. During the last century, every five to ten years a new brow trend has emerged, from thin and round to thick and arched. Today brows are more natural, but well groomed. There is no eyebrow trend or rule about how they should look. Every one of us is born with our own brow style; the hair grows differently in every one of us.

But it's good to know where brows should start and end (see the photo). Any hair outside that line, you (or your esthetician) should pluck. The best way to get your best brows is to see an esthetician, who will clean and shape them on the first visit. Thereafter, you can do it yourself. That way you won't have any mistakes on your brows (too thin, a funny shape, or holes).

I like beautiful eyebrows, but they don't necessarily have to be the most perfect or always be filled, especially in the daytime. Overly groomed and filled brows look unnatural. Keep them real.

When your eyebrows are misshapen and do not flow smoothly, the perspective of your face is thrown off. Rather than noticing your face as a whole, viewers cannot focus their eyes on one place, particularly when viewing you eye to eye. You'd be surprised at how much more intently someone will listen to you when you have perfect brows.

# TECHNIQUES

**GINA VELTRI** *at Tracey & Byron Salon, Beverly Hills, CA, a sought-after eyebrow guru whose clients include many Hollywood A-list actors*

## Waxing

With wax there is a lot of pulling on the delicate skin around the eye. When the hairs are pulled in the opposite direction from the natural growth pattern, they end up unmanageable and out of control when they grow back. Mistakes are made with wax more than with any other technique, I find. Waxing is also limited as to the shape you can achieve. Waxing leaves the skin around the brow area shiny and unnatural looking, especially when you put on makeup. One wrong slip of the wax may leave you in danger of permanently damaging the hair follicles.

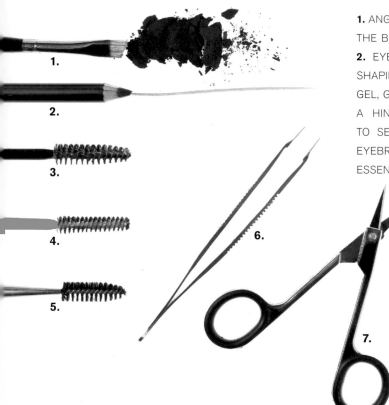

**1.** ANGLED EYEBROW BRUSH, FOR FILLING THE BROWS WITH A MATTE EYE SHADOW **2.** EYEBROW PENCIL, FOR FILLING AND SHAPING THE BROWS **3.** TINTED BROW GEL, GOOD FOR FAIR BROWS TO PROVIDE A HINT OF COLOR **4.** EYEBROW GEL, TO SET TOO-LONG OR WILD BROWS **5.** EYEBROW BRUSH **6.** TWEEZERS, AN ESSENTIAL **7.** CUTICLE SCISSORS, FOR CUTTING THE BROWS

## Threading

This is probably the most painful and least precise method. What I find amazing about threading is that it can literally grab every tiny little hair. Some find the technique very painful. I can often tell when someone has had her brows threaded because she is left with what looks like two straight lines above her eyes. The tip of the arch, which is the highest point of the brow, is often removed.

## Tweezing

I prefer tweezing, as it is the least painful method and gives you the most control and more options, and the hair does not grow back as quickly or erratically as with waxing. Tweezing leaves you with the least possibility of irritation. With the proper technique, tweezing can be almost painless. Without exaggeration, seven out of ten people fall asleep in my chair! What I can achieve with tweezers is limitless. Oftentimes I have a client who comes in and says, "I was told I could never have this shape brow" and my answer to that is "Yes, you can." I spend a half hour with each client, shaping her brows hair by hair.

### How often should I see my esthetician?

Once a month, if possible. There are always exceptions; some clients need to come in every three weeks, and some can stretch it to five or six weeks.

### Will the hairs stop growing over time if I keep plucking?

Some areas of the brow are much more prone to follicle damage than others. That's why it's important to follow the strict rules of a professional. My mantra is "When in doubt, don't pull it out!"

### What is the biggest mistake made when shaping brows?

Overtweezing. That's when people tweeze too much from between the brows, leaving them overspaced, or tweeze too much from the ends of the brows. Those are danger zones because they are prone to follicle damage. Also, due to age, hormones, or even a thyroid condition, women may lose hair at the ends of their brows. I cannot stress how important it is to be very careful with that area. I can always tell if someone is right- or left-handed by her tweezing pattern. For

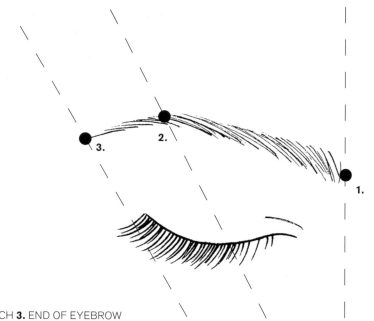

**1.** START **2.** ARCH **3.** END OF EYEBROW

example, if you are right-handed it is usually your left brow that is overtweezed. When using your crossover hand (tweezer in your right hand crossing over your face to tweeze your left brow), all too often you lose perspective and overtweeze. *Do not be a habitual picker!* You do not need to tweeze your brows every day. This applies to everyone! Do not clean up your own brows any more than every three days. And beware of magnifying mirrors. If a hair cannot be seen with your own naked eye, chances are no one else will see it either.

## How to Tweeze

Invest in an inexpensive pair of straight-edge cuticle scissors, a twirler brush (looks like a mascara brush), and a decent pair of tweezers. Start by brushing the hairs up with the twirler brush and trimming the long hairs. Make sure not to cut too closely. With a slanted shadow liner brush and brow powder, fill the brow in to the desired shape (forget those silly stencils) and tweeze the excess hair outside the desired shape. Look at pictures in magazines to get some ideas of good shapes. Be realistic about your own brows and those in a picture that you are hoping to duplicate. Be conservative.

### What can I do if my eyebrows are superfair?

A quick fix is tinted brow gel and/or filling your brows in with a light brown powder. Otherwise, I suggest having a professional tint your brows.

### How about bleaching the brows?

This is common on photo shoots because it gives the makeup artist more room to play with makeup, but it is also common in real life. Lightening the brows is very common—every day women bleach their brows—but I suggest having it done by a professional so you do not turn your eyebrows orange. I also feel that an experienced brow professional gives a much better result than your hair colorist can. The best result comes when I bleach the brows with a 10 to 20 volume peroxide and bleaching powder combination. Sometimes that is enough, but if the hair is too yellow-looking, I add ash-tone hair dye for just a few seconds to take away the yellowness.

## Eyebrow Tattooing

I am generally not for tattooing the brows. However, a few professionals are skilled at it. Spot filling can be helpful for women with thin brows. Again, it depends on the professional. An important thing to remember when considering tattooing a full brow is that often the person performing this service is not up on the proper shape. Also, as we age the face falls, but that does not mean everything falls evenly and symmetrically. Once your brows are permanently tattooed, you lose the option to "cheat" the brows symmetrically. Brows usually have to be tattooed every two years, depending on your coloring. A darker pigment will hold longer than one that is lighter. Make sure to look at many before-and-after pictures. Commonly I see the pigment turn dark blue or green. Again, though, I know some highly experienced professionals who do remarkable work.

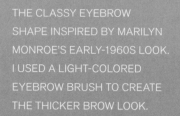

## Eyebrow Gel

I call this the icing on the cake. Gel can finish the brows off to perfection. I always end a brow-shaping session with gel. Brow gel can also be helpful to keep the brows tame between shaping appointments. Also, when you fill in the brow with powder or pencil, the gel helps to lock in the color. I often go without makeup; however, I always have my brows filled in perfectly. I fill them in with brow powder and follow with clear brow gel, and the color stays all day. Even at the gym, through the toughest of workouts or sweating, they remain perfect without any dripping, smearing, or running.

Men, just like women, should groom their brows. I use the term "groom" as opposed to "shape." I start by trimming their brows, followed by tweezing. I am careful not to make them "perfect" in any way, often leaving hairs out of line. I am not a proponent of waxing in general, but when it comes to a man's brows I really must say no! Commonly men's brows are left too sharp and shaped by waxing. A man's brows should look tidy and not "done"—unless he's performing in drag, of course.

### How about Asian brows? They usually grow downhill.

Yes, they do—the outer half, at least. I start by brushing the brows up to trim them and then brush the outer half down and trim them underneath. On the whole, Asian brows are not dense, so proceed with caution when tweezing.

### What do you prefer, eyebrow pencil or matte eye shadow, to fill your brows?

Generally, I prefer matte eye shadow, and it is what I most commonly use. When asked by clients what they should use, I say it is up to them. The end result is the same; it is just a matter of what tool they feel more comfortable using.

### Any tricks for the 50+ age group?

For many, a professional brow shaping can give the appearance of an instant face-lift! I mean this in the best way possible. However, as we age it is very important to take the arch down. After a certain age, a brow that is highly arched can actually be aging. I often tell a client to look at childhood/baby pictures of themselves for guidance.

### What is your favorite era of eyebrow trends, and why?

That's a tough question. I have so many favorites, simply because they go along with the overall look of that time. I must say, I like where we are today. There is no one "best" brow. I take in your overall look, your profession, your personality, and your lifestyle and decide what's the best for you and your face. No hard and fast rules! We are all individuals with our own individual brows!

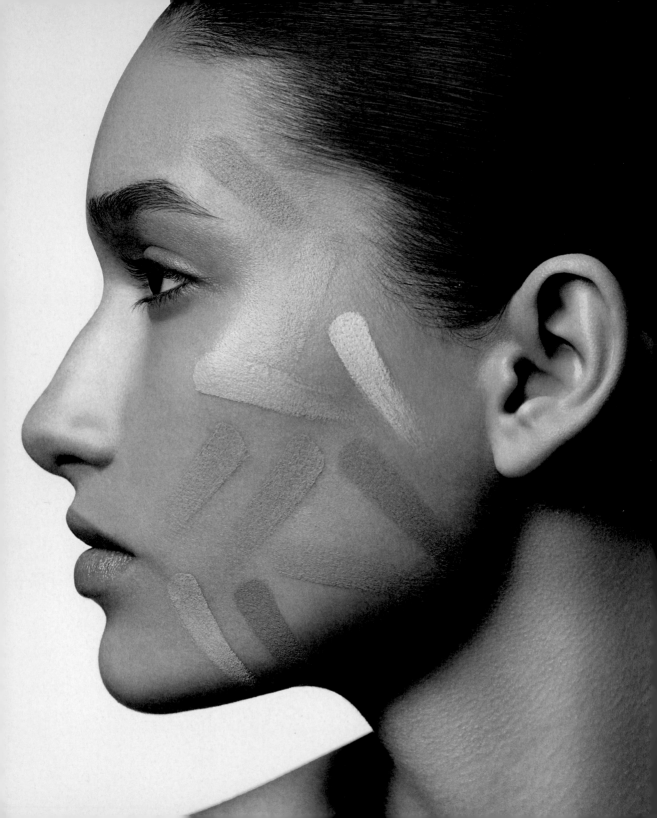

# 11 FOUNDATIONS AND BASES

**The right foundation looks and feels light. It should never look as though you are wearing makeup. You can get two or three different colors of the same brand and mix them to get the perfect shade. Foundation is not a skin care product. Even after you choose the base for your skin type, you will still need a moisturizer with SPF 15 to 20 or sunblock and an eye-area cream.**

My favorite place to buy makeup is at a department store, because it has everything in one place.

## CONSIDER FUNCTION AND LIFESTYLE

Ask yourself, "Why do I need a base? Is it for everyday use, is it for evening makeup only, is it for my resort vacation, or is it something else? Do I want more coverage, or do I just want to achieve a dewy look? Or do I want a totally matte finish?"

## TINTED MOISTURIZER

For the most natural result, use a tinted moisturizer, which makes the skin look light and natural. If you need to cover something, such as darker inner eye corners or a pimple, use a concealer on top of the tinted moisturizer. This is the favorite product of many makeup artists. It's also great for a dewy look.

**Light coverage:** Liquid foundation. Great for daytime. Also available in an oil-free formulation.

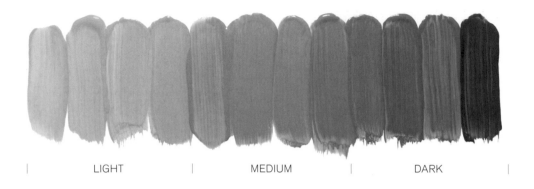

| | | | | |
|---|---|---|---|---|
| | LIGHT | | MEDIUM | DARK |

**Medium coverage:** Cream liquid foundation. The texture is creamier and "heavier" and covers the skin totally but still somewhat naturally. Semimatte and matte finishing. Good for evenings when your makeup must be perfectly done. Also available in an oil-free formulation.

**Mousse:** Gives a semimatte or matte result, medium coverage. Light formulation that glides easily on the skin, thanks to silicon mixes.

**Cream-powder compact:** Great for touch-ups.

**Stick:** Very handy, and comes in light-to-medium coverage. Use it directly from the stick or with the help of a sponge.

**Spray foundation:** After the airbrush trend, some companies came up with a spray foundation formula. It's quite complicated to use, and many brands are way too cakey and drying. The application is not the handiest, though it might be the fastest.

**High-pigment cream base:** The most covering base. Great for theater productions or TV makeup, but way too heavy for everyday use. Use only if you need to cover a birthmark or a scar.

STILL LIFE: KIINO VILLAND

## HOW TO BUY FOUNDATION

Take your old base with you when shopping for a new one. Maybe you were happy with the old color but the formula was too thick, or the old one was the wrong color (too light, dark, ashy, yellow, pink). Maybe it was too dry for your skin type, maybe it was too oily, or maybe it provided too much pigmentation and coverage. Or perhaps it didn't cover enough. It's good to read the fashion and beauty magazines to catch up on the latest products and test them as well. And remember, what looks perfect on your best girlfriend won't necessarily look good on you. There will always be a new base product on the market, every month. But don't get confused; some of them are no better than the ones that have been available for years.

Don't wear any makeup while shopping for a new base product. Of course you can wear mascara and lipstick, but nothing else on your face.

Take your time and test different brands, ask questions, and if there is a makeup artist, ask her/him to do a test makeup with the product you think might be the right one. When you test on yourself, always test on your jawline. That way you will see how the foundation matches your neck and face.

Carry a hand mirror with you so you can step outside and test the color in natural light. There shouldn't be any shade differences. It should look like the perfect shade. If it's not, wipe it off and go on to the next. Never test foundation on the back of your hand because the skin on your hands is either lighter or darker than that on your face.

All cosmetic brand representatives want to sell their own product by telling you their product is the best. And sometimes it's true. But look around and test. Many of today's base products have SPF 8 to 20 and antiaging ingredients to smooth your lines.

---

*TIP  If your base gets dry and cakey during the day, spray Evian water on your face (for just a few seconds, from a distance) and blend the base with the help of a sponge. Don't add more powder, because it will just make the skin look drier. And remember to drink plenty of water.*

---

## HOW TO APPLY FOUNDATION

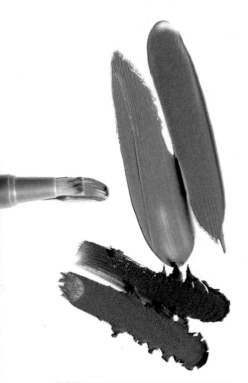

DIFFERENT TYPES OF CONCEALER

1. Start with a clean face.

2. Add your daily moisturizer and/or a primer or sunblock alone.

3. Put a drop of foundation on the palm of your hand and tap the foundation brush or a triangle sponge on the foundation. If you use two or three different fluids, mixing them to match your skin tone, this is when to mix them.

4. There is no rule as to where you should start the foundation application, but I like to start in on the cheeks. Go all over your face, remembering the eyelids and lips as well. Apply the foundation evenly. Be extra careful on the T-zone, where makeup tends to fade during the day.

5. Brush with quick and short strokes all over your face and, using the sponge, tap the fluid lightly onto your skin. Blend it well.

6. Finish the application on your jawline and blend the foundation well, fading to the neck.

Now it's time for concealer—or maybe not. Many times you don't need any more coverage because the liquid foundation or tinted moisturizer has already made the skin even. But if you have dark circles under your eyes or in the inner corners, or brown spots or blemishes to cover up, now is the time for concealer. Light-reflecting pencil is a good choice for dark circles. Use a concealer brush. If your skin is dry or wrinkled around the eyes, choose a lighter, liquid concealer, which is more moisturizing than a creamier concealer. Don't cover the blemishes too much, because they actually will start showing much more. Just a simple tap with your fingertip right on the top of the blemish is enough. Remember to blend well! Powder your face. Be light-handed around the eyes if you have dry skin or the eye

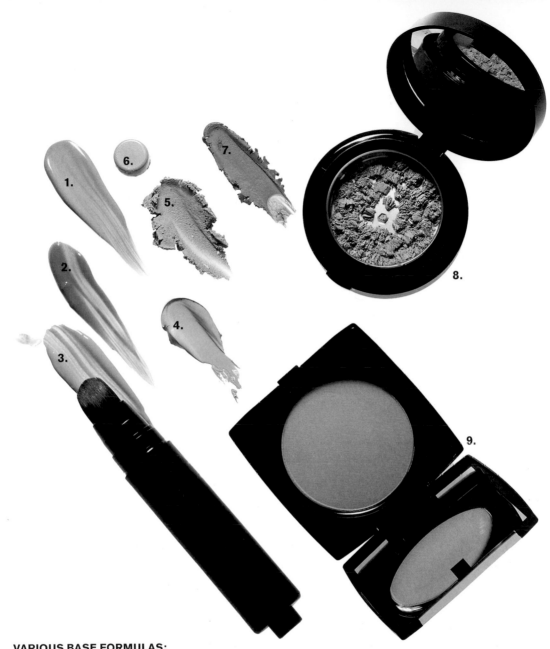

**VARIOUS BASE FORMULAS:**

**1.** TINTED MOISTURIZER **2.** GEL-BASED TINTED MOISTURIZER **3.** LIQUID FOUNDATION WITH AN AUTOMATIC BRUSH **4.** HIGH-PIGMENTATION CREAM BASE **5.** MOUSSE FOUNDATION **6.** STICK FOUNDATION **7.** CREAM-POWDER FOUNDATION **8.** MINERAL POWDER BASE **9.** COMPACT POWDER FOUNDATION (WORKS ON DRY OR DAMP SPONGE)

area is wrinkled. But you do need a little bit of powder to set the base. You can tap a hint of loose powder under the eyes with an eye shadow brush.

Sometimes testers in stores might not be clean and hygienic, so you can ask the cosmetics department representative to open a new product as a tester. It's also good to carry some tissue with you so you can wipe the base products off your skin when testing them.

*TIP  Did you know that you actually also pay more for big-label foundations than if the same product were packed in a simple plastic (recycled) bottle without a container? Don't get me wrong, there are fantastic products with fantastic containers, but this is good to remember. In the end, the big fashion labels create the illusion of being superfashionable with their packaging. Sometimes you can find the same ingredients in a less expensive brand.*

## PRIMERS

Primers make the skin look and feel much smoother. Primers create a barrier between the skin and foundation, and some of them contain light-reflecting ingredients.

Apply primer on top of your moisturizer; allow time for the moisturizer to be absorbed before applying the primer. A primer creates the perfect canvas for foundation to stay on your skin longer. It fills in fine lines, makes pores invisible, keeps the skin looking matte longer, and makes the skin look and feel really silky. It's a great product, especially for 30+ skin.

Some primers contain SPF 15 to 20; some are mattifying or hydrating. Make sure you get the right product for your skin type. Remember to apply a sunscreen under the primer if your foundation doesn't contain SPF/UVA/UVB.

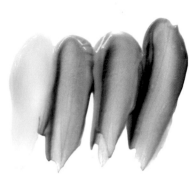

PRIMERS, AVAILABLE IN TRANSPARENT
OR COLOR-CORRECTING FORMULAS

## Color-Correcting Primers

These are really good and even out the skin tone. Use as a primer under your base.

**Green:** Reduces redness (amazing for those of you who have redness on the face)
**Apricot:** Warms the skin and counteracts discoloration
**Lavender:** Brightens dull or sallow skin

## Concealers

These cover the dark areas under and at the inner corners of your eyes. They mask any redness and color differences and render a pimple less noticeable. Use concealer after you apply foundation, because many times you don't need the concealer after the base is applied. Or you might need much less. Good concealer covers lightly and is not drying. I like silicon concealers that glide onto the skin smoothly. My absolute favorite is the pencil one with a brush. Use the following for your skin color:

**Fair skin:** A warm peach-toned concealer (yellow base)
**Deeper skin tones:** Orange-to-yellow undertone concealers work well

I always warm the concealer with my fingers in the palm of my hand. It helps it blend into the skin better and faster.

## Light-Reflecting Pencils

YSL was the first to introduce the new makeup tool Touche Éclat, a light-reflecting pencil, and soon afterward all the major brands had similar versions of this magic pencil, which lightens dark under-eye circles by adding light and lifting the eye area. I love to use this product, especially on those 40+. I apply it on top of a tinted moisturizer or liquid foundation and blend it well. I use just a bit of powder on top of the base; otherwise the eye area gets too shiny and oily-looking. I don't use light-reflecting pencils for highlighting the cheeks or other areas of the face. I like to use cream sticks or powder formats for that purpose.

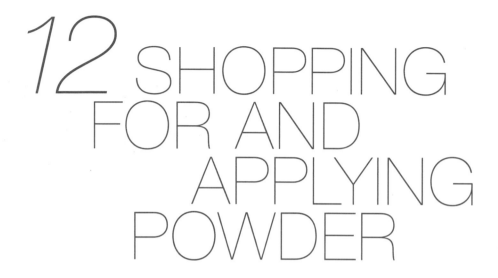

# 12 SHOPPING FOR AND APPLYING POWDER

**Powder is one of the oldest of all beauty products and is used by both women and men. It remains one of the most popular and highest selling items in the world of cosmetics.**

Powder keeps your skin and makeup matte, helps the rest of your makeup settle more smoothly on your face, and keeps it lasting longer. Powder is an important product for combination and oily skin because it absorbs oil. Color is the key to selecting the right powder for you. Fair skin is the easiest because you can use a transparent powder, but medium and dark skin colors need more attention when making color choices. The wrong color choice, just as with foundations, can make your skin appear too ashy, yellow, or red. Buy powder at the same time as foundation for the best results.

Sometimes I like a dewy look with almost no powder, sometimes I like a semidewy look, and sometimes the skin has to be all matte. Dry skin needs hardly any powder. For combination skin I apply more powder on the T-zone, and for oily skin I use powder all over the face. But powder is useful for all skin types as a way to set the foundation, and it also keeps eye shadows and liners on the eyes without looking smudgy.

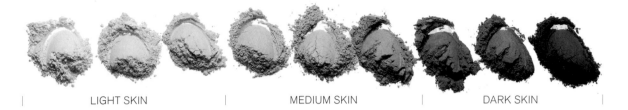

|  LIGHT SKIN  |  |  MEDIUM SKIN  |  |  DARK SKIN  |

**THE COLOR VARIATIONS OF LOOSE POWDERS**

For those 40+, be very light-handed with powders. You need the powder to set the base, but pay attention, especially around the eyes, where the skin is more dry and wrinkled. Too much powdering will inevitably bring out the crow's feet, fine lines, and wrinkles.

A powder puff is the best, and my all-time favorite, tool for applying loose powder. You can really press the powder onto the skin with the puff. The right technique is to take a small amount of loose powder from the container and tip it onto the palm of your hand; then press the puff onto the powder, swirl it on the hand, and start the application by tapping the powder all over your face, including your eyelids and lips (if your lips are very dry, skip this).

A brush is also a great tool for applying powder to your face, but you'll get a much lighter result. The technique is the same, but after you swirl the brush on the palm of your hand, you need to tap the powder brush so it doesn't hold too much product. Then start tapping the brush all over your face, very lightly, on the top of your base. This is the best technique, great for drier skin that needs less powder.

Compact powders and blotting papers are great for touch-ups. I like to use the papers first and then, if needed, add a little more powder on the needed area, such as nose, cheeks, chin, and forehead. If you simply add more and more powder during the day, your skin will start to look chalky.

STILL LIFE: KIINO VILLAND

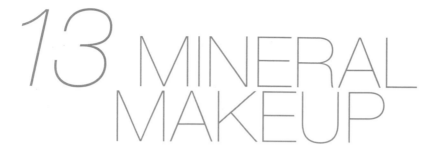

# 13 MINERAL MAKEUP

**Mineral makeup products have taken the cosmetics world by storm. You can buy products from big cosmetics brands, from online companies, or from TV vendors. Or you can make your very own blends in your kitchen.**

Mineral makeup is good, but don't be fooled by the words on the label. You must know what real benefits it provides.

As the name suggests, mineral makeup is made mostly of all-natural, finely ground minerals from the earth. They were already in use in ancient times, when people painted their bodies with earthy colors. But the real commercial boost for mineral makeup started in the mid-1970s, and then again in the mid-1990s. Today every major brand includes makeup in its selection.

The most common ingredients in the most popular brands are titanium dioxide, zinc oxide, silk mica, and hydrated silica. I prefer regular liquid foundations (ultrasheer formulas) or tinted moisturizers because I feel I get the most natural result with those formulations. Mineral makeup powder foundation is no better than a regular liquid foundation or tinted moisturizer. But again, for some, mineral makeup works perfectly.

**Mineral makeup is good if:**

- Your skin is young, 20+, without any serious blemishes to cover up.
- You have very sensitive skin or you have cosmetic allergies or rosacea (more than 14 million people suffer from rosacea in the United States alone).
- You have acne (mineral makeup might be the right product for you to cover up the areas and get more even-looking skin).
- You require hypoallergenic products because they don't contain fragrances, dyes, chemicals, or preservatives, so they shouldn't create irritation and rashes.
- You desire a natural look; the look is quite natural, and often just one single application in the morning lasts all day.
- You want to avoid clogging your pores.

## CONCERNS ABOUT MINERAL MAKEUP

Mineral makeup products are often labeled "all natural" and "pure." But be aware that that could mean a number of things. Mineral ingredients include mica (a light reflector that reduces fine lines and fills pores), titanium dioxide (provides a sunscreen and high coverage), and zinc oxide (provides sun protection and calms irritated skin), which have been used in "regular" foundations for years.

Bismuth oxychloride is an ingredient that gives some mineral makeup a glow. But be aware that it can also give you rashes and cystic acne.

Mineral makeup dries the skin, something to consider especially for the 40+ group. And because mineral makeup also gives a glow, your lines will be doubly visible. As a professional I prefer to use tinted moisturizer or a light liquid foundation and loose powder to build up a long-lasting, traditional base. Using the regular base, you apply the foundation on the eyelids and lips as well, and you get a longer-lasting base for eye and lip makeups.

Some mineral makeup products make darker skin tones look too ashy. I also don't recommend mineral makeup for oily skin. It may look good on you first thing in the morning, but during the day the oil starts to push through the makeup and the skin looks messy. Then you have to apply more mineral makeup, and you start to look like a cook with too much flour on her face. Some formulas include absorbing ingredients such as kaolin clay. But they don't help much. Stick with an oil-free primer, oil-free foundation, loose powder, and blotting paper combination.

### 100% Pure Silk Makeup

The best mineral makeup ingredient, 100% pure silk is one of the purest ingredients. It has many positive effects.

- It moisturizes the skin by sealing moisture into the skin. This is great, especially in dry weather!
- It entraps oil.
- It heals the skin after sun- and windburns.
- It has UV-blocking properties (because silk is meant to protect the silkworm, so those qualities should be present).
- It balances the skin's pH. Silk, in cosmetics generally, leaves the skin very smooth and literally silky, thanks to the amino acids (from non-animal-protein sources) it contains.

There are only a few mineral makeup companies that use 100% silk in their products.

## HOW TO APPLY MINERAL MAKEUP

You need a smaller powder brush, round shape blush brush, or Kabuki brush that comes with the most popular brands. Make sure the brush is made of real hair.

Sprinkle a dash of mineral powder (you need to apply very little powder; too much will give too much coverage and leave you glowing like the moon) on the inside of the container's lid and swirl the brush in the powder. Tap excess powder off the brush against the side of the lid and start the application. Use the brush on your skin in a circular motion all around your face, including the eyelids.

Be very light-handed around the eye area, especially if you have any lines and wrinkles; they will show up quite easily.

Concealer also comes in powder format. Apply it on top of the base, with the help of a smaller mineral makeup concealer brush on the areas where you need more coverage, such as the inner corners of the eyes or blemishes.

### Does mineral makeup also come in liquid foundations?

Yes, but real mineral makeup is always in powder form. If you are looking for a purer makeup product, stay with the powders.

### Can I sleep with mineral makeup on my face?

No. You should never sleep with any makeup on. Always wash your face before you go to bed. Mineral makeup is a makeup product, not a skin care product.

### How do I wash mineral makeup off my face?

Just like any other makeup, using a cleanser that is appropriate for your skin type. Cleansing oil is the best. If your skin is oily, use a foam cleanser and a toner that will double-cleanse the pores. I highly recommend using a toner after the cleanser to make sure you get everything off. The toner also prepares your skin for the serum and/or cream.

### Is mineral makeup water-resistant?

Yes, many of them are water-resistant.

### Some mineral makeup contains SPF 15; does it really work?

Sure it works, but I would use 15 to 30 SPF with UVA and UVB protection under the mineral makeup, because during the day you might forget to apply more mineral makeup and then you won't have the protection anymore.

### Mineral makeup is drying on my skin, but I love the product. What can I do?

Apply a good moisturizer with SPF 15 to 30 with UVA and UVB protection under the mineral makeup. Let the skin absorb the moisturizer completely before applying the makeup. But if your skin is superdry, the result will look way too dry; instead use a day cream and a tinted moisturizer on top of that. No powder is needed. For oily skin, use a purifying toner and oil-free moisturizer (keeps your skin matte) before applying the mineral makeup. This combination will keep the skin matte for a longer time. And don't forget to have oil blotting papers with you all the time, and use them before you add more mineral makeup.

---

*TIP* *What you see on TV shopping channels doesn't always look good in real life. It's really hard to buy any makeup from TV because you can't test the products and shades in natural light.*

---

### Does mineral makeup work for deeper skin tones?

There are quite a few mineral makeup companies that specialize in deeper skin tones. You just must research and try them on your skin. You can always ask the artist at the makeup counter to try a mineral makeup base on you. And always step out into natural light to check out the result.

### Isn't the application quite messy?

You must practice the application. The powder might fly at first. The new modern mineral makeups are packed in handy grinder compacts that are less messy than before. Apply the mineral base before you dress up to avoid getting the makeup on your clothes. Mineral makeup application is pretty fast in the end. Once you get the hang of it, you can be done in just a few minutes.

### What about other mineral makeup products: eye shadows, eyeliners, blushes, and lipsticks?

This is tricky. There are hundreds of products out there that are labeled as mineral makeup, and most of them contain only 2 to 5 percent of mineral ingredients; it's all about marketing and how companies try to make you buy more and more cosmetics. The real mineral eye shadows and blushes are in powder form. Lipsticks and glosses are sometimes saturated with mineral pigments, and some of them have shea butter to smooth out the product. You can create your own colored lip balm by dipping a lip balm into a pink blush powder, for example, and get a beautiful and natural result. Or you can make a lip gloss using Vaseline and blush; just mix them together and apply to your lips. Mineral eyeliners come in a powdery format as well: you dip a wet eyeliner brush into the powder, mix the powder and water together on the palm of your hand, and apply.

There are also mineral mascaras, nail polishes, eyebrow pencils, kohls, and lip liners that contain mineral pigments.

### Can one be allergic to mineral makeup?

There are so many different levels of sensitivities and allergies. If you think you are allergic to mineral makeup or any other makeup, simply quit using the product. You should also get allergy-tested to learn exactly which ingredient is causing the reaction. The most common causes are perfumes and dyes.

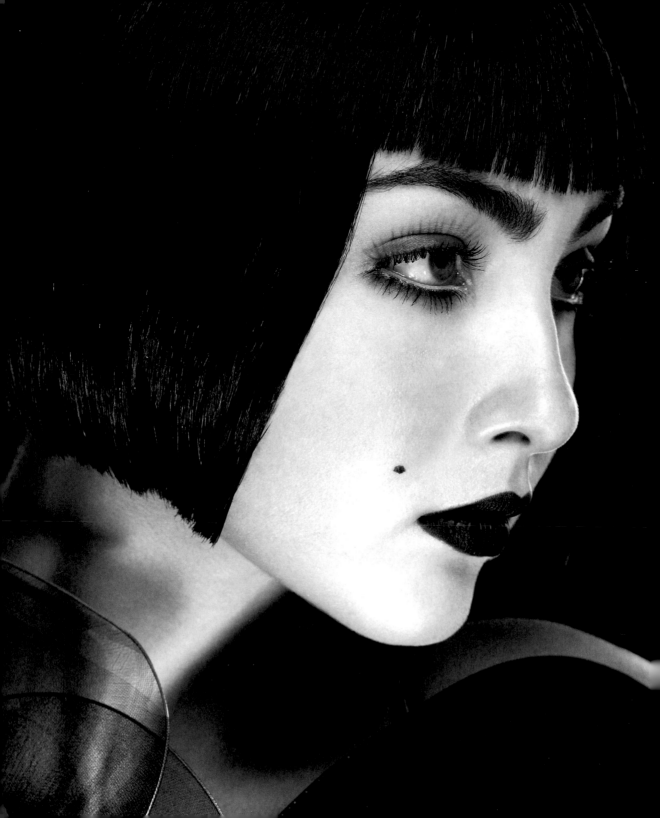

# 14 EYES

PHOTO: GIULIANO BEKOR/MODEL: SCARLET @ ELITE/HAIR: CHRISTIAN MARC/STYLING: VANESSA GELDBACH

**Eye makeup is all about the lashes, which give your eye shape and depth. It's no surprise, then, that mascara usually ranks as number one or two, right after lipstick, as the most popular product for women.**

The first mascara was made by Eugène Rimmel in the 1830s. He was inspired by an old Arabian henna powder trick for the lashes. The more modern version of mascara was developed in 1913 by the chemist T. L. Williams, who made mascara for his sister Mabel (the beginning of the Maybelline cosmetic brand). In the 1930s, Houbigant's cake mascara was very popular in Europe. But it was the cosmetics mogul Helena Rubinstein who created the revolutionary tube mascara with a wand. Since then, there have been hundreds of mascaras on the market, and every month a new mascara is born, it seems.

### What does mascara do?
Mascara is used to darken, thicken, emphasize, lengthen, and/or define the lashes.

### What is mascara made of?
The base is wax and dye or pigment.

### How do I choose the best brush?
The brush is the key to a great lash look. Small brushes with small bristles dye the lashes the best, because the smaller the brush, the better the dye catches onto the roots. Then again, longer bristles separate the lashes better. So get a combination of the two. Curved brushes do curl the lashes a little, but you actually need to curl your lashes with a professional eyelash curler before applying mascara.

MASCARA IS USED TO DARKEN,
THICKEN, EMPHASIZE, LENGTHEN,
AND/OR DEFINE THE LASHES.

### Which mascara is the best for me?

Your lifestyle and uses determine the mascara you should choose. Will you use it on an everyday basis? Does it need to last through your yoga class? If your lashes are short, you may want a lengthening mascara. If your lashes are superlong, you may prefer a more separating mascara. Are you going on a long-awaited vacation to a beautiful resort? You may want to find a water-resistant blue-turquoise mascara. Read the beauty magazines, especially the ones that test different mascaras. When you find your favorite, it will become your best friend in your makeup bag!

### What is tubing mascara?

It is a mascara formal that was created in Japan in the late 1990s. It comes in tubes and has a flexible polymer that is a great film former. It gives you just the dye, nothing else. You rinse the mascara off your lashes with warm water. It's a good option when you need your mascara to last through rain, shine, and activity.

### How do I curl my lashes?

Marlene Dietrich used a teaspoon to curl her lashes, but I prefer a professional eyelash curler. Position the curler as close as possible to the roots of your lashes. Keeping your eyes open, gently squeeze the curler closed. Pump the curler once to see if the lashes are curled enough. If not, do it again. If your eyes are wide and the curler is too small, you can use a so-called corner curler, which will curl the rest of the lashes that have been left out. I also like a heating curler. It gets its energy from a small 1.5-volt battery. Wait a couple of minutes for the brush to heat, and add mascara. Place the brush on the lashes, flex the lashes with the brush, wait three or four seconds, and release the brush, and your lashes will be beautifully curled. It's really easy.

### Can I curl my lashes after I have applied mascara?

No. If you curl lashes when they are still wet, they will stick to the curler and might break. Even if you wait until the lashes are dry, they might break. And because you already have applied the mascara and given the lashes a dry coverage, they won't curl as beautifully as when you do it before applying the mascara.

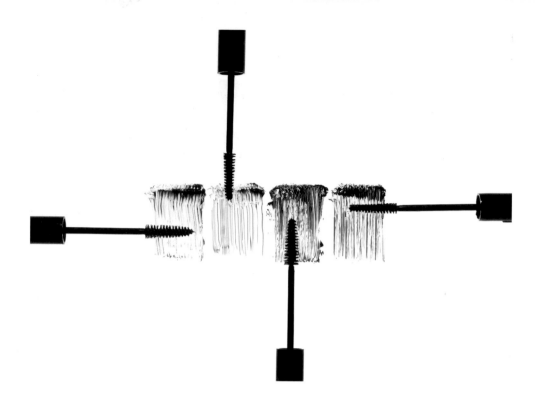

### Can mascara actually lengthen or thicken the lashes?

Some mascaras contain rayon or nylon fibers and actually do lengthen the lashes, because mascara clings to the lashes like miniextensions. But don't expect a miracle; it's a very small change. The thickening/volumizing mascaras have a thicker formula of waxes and silicone polymers that, together with their bigger and thicker brush, coat the lashes and make them appear bulkier.

### How much mascara should I apply?

One to three coats. By applying one coat, you will get a very beautiful and natural lash look. The second coat will deepen the look, and the third coat will make a strong look. Remember that the more coats you add, the more the lashes separate, giving that "spider" lash look that was very popular and fashionable in the late 1960s and early 1970s. If you decide to apply two to three coats of mascara, make sure you comb the lashes in between with a metallic eyelash comb or brush the lashes with a clean lash brush. If you add more mascara after the lashes are dry, you will get a clumpy result. But sometimes that looks really cool!

### How about colored mascaras—blue, green, turquoise?

Black is the most popular and suits everyone. Brown is a great option if you are fair and your lashes are lighter; it gives a softer look. The colored ones—navy blue, shocking blue, green, turquoise—don't show as well on dark lashes as on lighter ones. Red and white might look cool too, but I would leave them for Halloween parties.

### When does mascara get old?

Two months from the second you start to use the mascara. It's very important to change your mascara every sixty days. Mascara gathers bacteria that can be very harmful to your eyes. And never, ever lend your mascara to anyone, even your mother or best girlfriend. Mascara is a very personal makeup item, just like lipstick or lip liner. You never know if someone has an eye infection, and by lending your mascara it's 100 percent sure you will get pinkeye, too, if she has it.

### My lashes go straight even when I curl them before applying the mascara!

Try waterproof mascara, because it contains the waxes that are the most effective in keeping and holding the curves in place. Heat the curler's rubber part with a blow dryer; this helps the hair of the lashes to curl better, and the curl lasts longer, especially when used with waterproof mascara. Waterproof mascara calls for waterproof mascara remover. Without that it's very difficult and damaging to get the makeup off.

The other option is an eyelash perm. It lasts three months and should be done by a professional.

### I have sensitive eyes. Can I use mascara?

There are many mascara brands out there that are made especially for sensitive eyes or for people who wear contact lenses. These mascaras don't contain silicons, alcohol, perfumes, or lanolin that might irritate the eyes. Usually the ingredients are more organic, or at least they're trying to be.

### My mascara always smudges. What can I do?

You might have oily skin and eyelids. Water-resistant mascara should take care of that problem. Also, make sure you use an oily skin–type skin care program so that your skin will stay matte as long as possible. Use an oil-free base and loose powder on the eyelids when applying foundation; this will provide a good base for the eye makeup and prevent the mascara from smudging your lids. And always carry a survivor kit with you: a clean sponge, cream-powder foundation, and Q-tips.

### Should I pump mascara?

You should never pump a mascara wand too much because that will dry out your mascara very quickly. One pump is sufficient. So my advice is to pump once, blot the wand on tissue, and then apply the mascara on your lashes. After that use a lash comb, if needed. Do it right after you have finished the application, because once the mascara dries it's really difficult to separate the lashes.

## THE REMEDY FOR SHORT OR PALE LASHES

To make short lashes appear fuller, the key is not to make them longer at all; you should get almost the same length as your own natural lashes, and the result will look surprisingly natural. And you don't need to use mascara anymore, because the result will amaze you. The extensions won't damage your own lashes.

- You can use individual fake lashes that will give you help for that occasional day.
- A better option is to get eyelash extensions. Today's extensions are safe, and you can swim, play sports, and even enjoy a spa and sauna without worrying that they will fall off. The lashes are synthetic, and the result is very natural. The process of applying takes up to two hours. The lashes last about four to six weeks and cost $150 to $350. The extensions will last longer if you don't use eye makeup remover or oil-based cleansers and don't touch or scrub your eyes (if you have allergies, this might be a habit for you).
- Eyelash growth gel will help your own lashes grow thicker and longer. Use it twice a day, morning and evening, on the roots of your lashes for

28 days straight, and then once a day. One of the ingredients that stimulates eyelash growth is soy lecithin liposome. You can use the gel even while wearing contact lenses.

## COLORING YOUR LASHES

If your lashes are very fair, dyeing the lashes is one option. This is great if you play a lot of sports, especially swimming. It's also good if you don't have time for makeup. (See chapter 18, "Three-Minute-a-Day Makeup.") Don't ever dye your lashes yourself, for safety reasons. Always go to a professional hair and beauty salon. The color will last 4 to 6 weeks.

*Famous Mascara Queens* Joan Crawford in her 1930s MGM portraits, Twiggy's 1960s lash look, Liza Minnelli's 1970s spider-eye makeup, and Madonna, whose lashes are the key to her look.

## FAKE EYELASHES

There are so many different kinds to choose from. Make sure you know what you want before you go to the beauty supply shop. Basic lashes are made of synthetics or human hairs. Some companies make lashes of mink hair that look amazing, especially for evening makeup. Use white (clear) or black adhesive. I personally like black, because it allows me to see the result faster (white takes a minute or two to become clear). There is no rule as to whether mascara should be applied before fake lashes or after. If I use individual lashes, I add mascara beforehand, because that way it's much easier to see how the lashes set and separate, and then I can easily find the spots where the individuals need to be placed. Sometimes I don't use mascara after adding the individuals if I want a more natural look. To add depth, mascara is needed.

**A single individual lash** gives the most natural look. Add them in the middle of the natural separation of your lashes, on the roots of the lash line. Dip each lash into an adhesive with tweezers. You can start in the middle or the outer corner, whatever feels best. Even three individuals make a difference. I usually add four to six individuals per eye.

**Cluster individuals** are more popular than single lashes because they're easier to add and you can see the result faster. You can choose from short, medium, and long ones. Color options are black or brown.

**Natural-size,** daytime false lashes. Make a thin pencil or liquid eyeliner line at the roots of the lashes before adding the fake lashes. It hides the strip, and the effect is more natural. Try the lashes on your eyes before adding the adhesive; the strip might be too long, and if so you should cut it shorter. Use the other end of the eyeliner brush to add the adhesive to the strip, wait five seconds, and start putting the lashes on the lash line, starting from the outer, middle, or inner corners of the eyes. Help the process along with the eyeliner handle. Blink your eyes and check that the fake lashes are properly set.

## EYE PENCIL AND LINER

Liners are a very classy way to emphasize the eyes and give instant depth to your look, whether a narrow liquid eyeliner line or a deeper and darker dramatic smudged eye pencil/kohl combination.

Gel formula stays longer and doesn't fall off during the day the way powder-format liners and matte eye shadows do. Many gel liners are water-resistant. Gel liners are easy to apply because they glide onto the lids easily. One of my favorite products is an automatic eyeliner pencil. Before you start lining your eyes, you should know the differences among the various tools.

### Eye Pencil

Great for all kinds of lining, from ultrasoft to ultrastrong, and are available in many colors: white, brown, black, purple, blue, green, gold, and more. They come in regular-

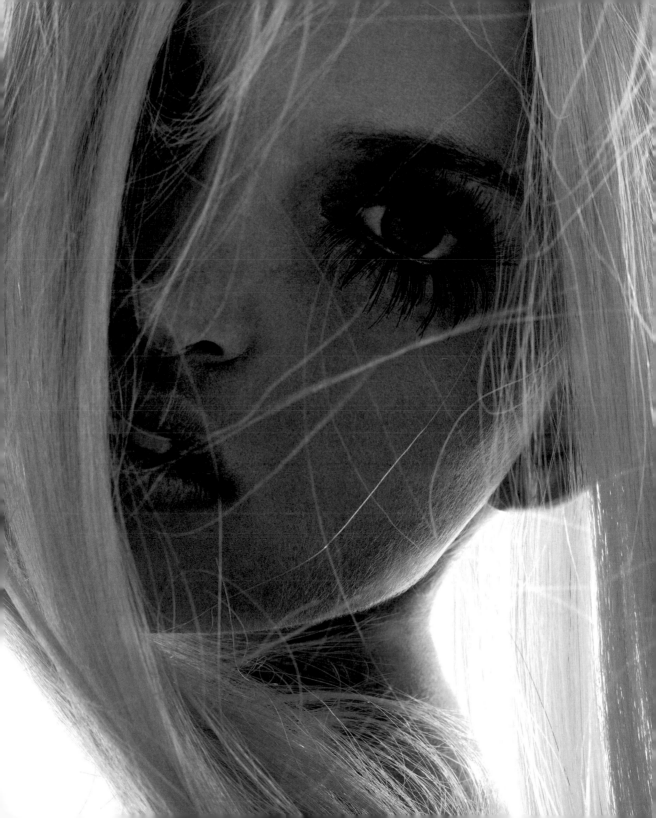

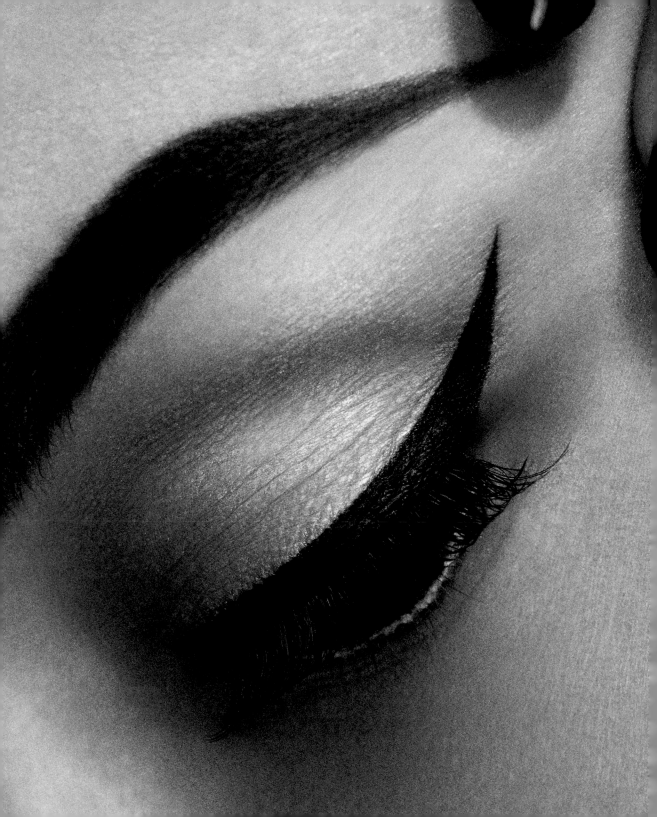

PHOTO: KURT ISWARIENKO/MODEL: JAIME @ NOUS MODELS/STILL LIFE: KIINO VILLAND

## FAKE LASHES FROM TOP TO BOTTOM:

1.  AN INDIVIDUAL AND A CLUSTER.
    GREAT FOR DAY AND EVENING LOOKS.

2.  NATURAL SIZE, GIVES DEPTH TO YOUR EYES.
    GOOD FOR DAYTIME.

3.  ONE OF MY FAVORITE ONES. OPENS UP THE EYES.
    GREAT FOR EVENING LOOKS.

4.  GREAT FOR THE '50s LOOK.

5.  CROSSING LASHES CREATE THE FULLNESS.

6.  GREAT FOR THE '30s LOOK.

7.  GREAT FOR THE '60s LOOK.

8.  GREAT FOR A MORE DRAMATIC '60s LOOK.

9.  GIVES MAXIMUM DEPTH TO THE EYES.
    GREAT FOR DRAMATIC EVENING MAKEUP.

10. GREAT FOR THE '70s LOOK.

11. BOTTOM LASHES FOR '60s AND '70s LOOKS.

and large-size pencils. I like the classic wooden pencils you can sharpen, because I have more control. Sometimes I need to work with a sharper tip and sometimes a rounder one. With some pencils, you twist the end out. The problem with those is that the tip gets too round and soft, and then it's really hard to get a good line. They are excellent for smoky eye makeup because you don't need to get a perfect line, just the color on the lash line (which you will smudge anyway). Pencils are also available in matte and shimmer/metallic formulas, and also in waterproof.

I store my pencils in the refrigerator, especially in the summertime. If it's warm, the wax can get too soft, and then it's hard to work with them (points break). The bathroom cabinet is also a good place for storage, because it's cool and dark.

## Kohl

This liner works the best inside the bottom and upper lids, giving an instant cat's-eye look. It is not great if you have small eyes because it shrinks the eyes a little; if so, you can use white kohl, which opens up the eyes. Black is the most common and popular color choice. You will need to touch up the liner during the day, so please make sure you carry the liner and a couple of Q-tips with you.

## White Inside Liner

This is a miracle worker that really opens your eyes and takes the eyes to another level. It's great for small eyes. Keep this pencil with you during the day as well. Check out page 260, about white inside liner.

## Eye Shadow

You can use matte eye shadow as a powder liner. Just tap a small no. 5 brush on the eye shadow and start lining the lash line. It gives a very natural result. Light brown, brown, dark brown, dark gray, and black are the most used colors, but you can do it with any color you desire.

## Liquid Liner

Use a matte eye shadow as a liquid liner. You need a no. 6 liquid eyeliner brush and a little water. Dip the tip of the brush into water and swirl the brush on the eye shadow long enough to get the color onto the brush. Mix the color on the palm of your hand before you start lining your eyes.

## Pencil Liner

Use an automatic pencil liner, which is really easy to use. The color lasts a long time, and the brush is designed to make very sharp lines.

PHOTO: RANDEE ST. NICHOLAS/MODEL: STEPHANIE @ NEXT/HAIR: LOUISE MOON/NAILS: JENNA HIPP

THIS EYE MAKEUP WAS DONE
BY USING BLACK KOHL TO GET
A MORE INTENSE LOOK.

ELECTRIC BLUE LOOKS GOOD
ON EVERY SKIN TONE. ALSO TRY
TURQUOISE AND BRIGHT GREEN.

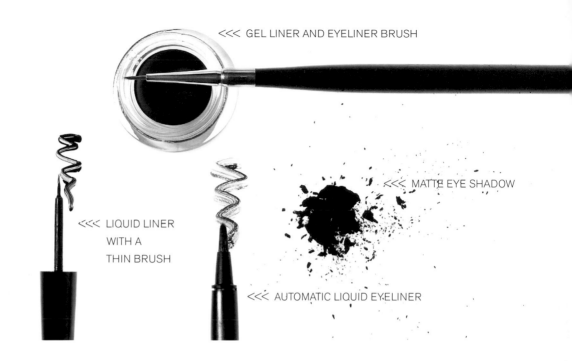

<<< GEL LINER AND EYELINER BRUSH

<<< MATTE EYE SHADOW

<<< LIQUID LINER
WITH A
THIN BRUSH

<<< AUTOMATIC LIQUID EYELINER

PHOTO: KURT ISWARIENKO/MODEL: ISABELLA @ LA MODELS/HAIR: LOUISE MCON. STILL LIFE: KIINO VILLAND

## Gel Eyeliner

This gives a smoother result than liquid liners do. It's easy to use and quite water-resistant.

### *How can I know which liner is the best for me?*

If you are new to lining your eyes, start with a pencil because it's much easier to practice with an eye pencil than a liquid liner. You will be blending the lines with a brush, anyway. Basic colors from brown to black are safe, but you can also try bolder ones, such as electric blue, deep green, purple, silver (opens up the eyes), or turquoise.

Gel-powder liners are great because you can fix them quite easily if you make any mistakes. They are available in many cool color choices.

The most challenging is liquid liner. Practice applying it on top of the gel-powder. That way you will get to know the shape of your eyes and your strongest and weakest points. Make sure that both eyes are lined the same (shape and thickness).

Start in the middle of the lash line. Line with small strokes toward the outer corner. Don't do the inside corner yet, but do the other eye half as well. That way you can make sure that the eyes will be symmetrical. Then do the inside corners.

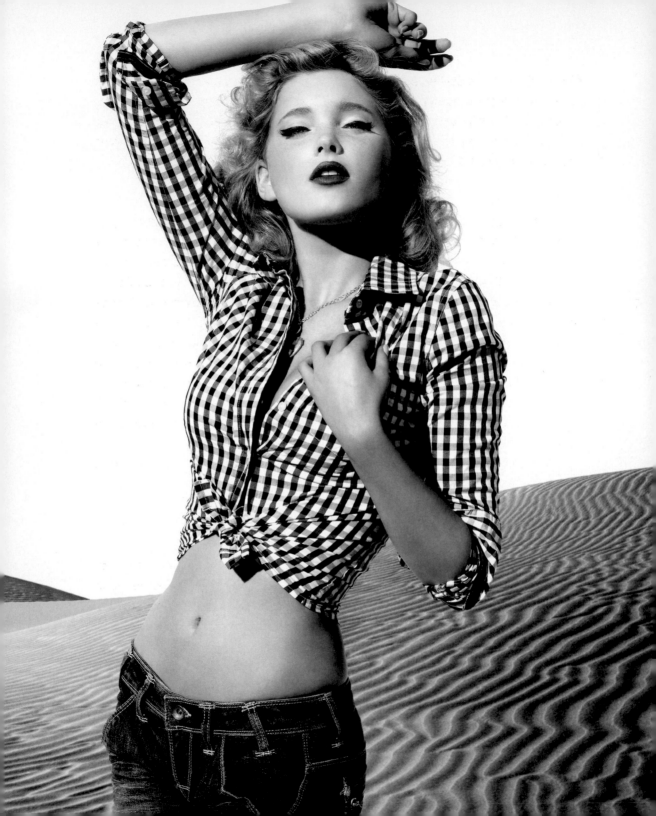

Depending on the desired style, you can make the whole line as thin as you want, or make the outer corners slightly thicker than the inside corners. This lifts the eyes and gives the elegant "cat's-eye" effect. You can also extend the liner like "wings" (see the photo), which creates a very glamorous look. I love liquid eyeliner, because it really gives that something extra to the eyes: allure and mystery.

### Why should I use a base on my eyelids before applying a liner?

It's okay to use pencil liner on bare skin, although I really recommend applying at least powder or tinted moisturizer plus powder to keep the liner in place. The problem is that the second you start sweating or your skin starts to get oily, your liner will melt and crack. This will happen sooner with a liquid eyeliner. So my advice is to prep the eyelids with a foundation or tinted moisturizer and loose powder. It's old school, but it works. There are also special eye base products that help liner and eye shadow stay on the lids longer. These are really great products, especially for women who have heavy eyelids or oily skin and have a hard time keeping the makeup in one place. Just add the product to clean, bare lids with your fingers, add foundation and powder, and start lining. Some brands don't tell you to add the foundation on top of the eyelid base product, just to powder the lids. Both ways work.

If you have oily skin, remember to use your skin-type toner in the morning to wipe extra oils off your skin, including the eyelids.

### Quick Fixes

Dip a Q-tip into water or eye makeup remover, press it between your fingers to remove the excess liquid, and wipe off the part of the liner that's off. Another good technique is to put a little liquid foundation on a Q-tip to wipe away the mistake. After the "mistake" is wiped off, tap foundation on carefully with the help of a concealer brush and finish with the powder.

Remember that the darker your skin is, the more pigment and color you can take. I love blues, turquoises, and metallic liners on dark and medium skin; fair skin can better take the most natural colors—light browns and gray—which look too washed out on darker skin tones. If you want a more natural look on darker skin, use dark gray or black, both of which look really good; black liner works for every skin color. For a more intense look, use black or dark gray liner and black mascara; this combination deepens the look of your eyes dramatically.

### Why doesn't my inside liner/kohl last very long on my eyes?

It's because the liner is applied to the inner rim of the eye and is touched by the tears in your eyes, which naturally takes kohl off the rim every time you blink. Some women have drier eyes, and their kohl stays on longer, whereas some have very watery eyes, and it's a challenge to keep the kohl in one place. So keep your kohl with you at all times for touch-ups during the day!

### How can I be sure if a liner is good quality?

Test it on your hand; the best pencils glide easily and aren't too soft (though they do break more easily) or too hard, in which case it's hard to get the color onto your lids. The best liquid liners are in pencil format; it's very much the brush design of the pencil as well as the ink that makes a great automatic liquid liner. The brush can't be too long and soft, or it will be really hard to get the lines even and thin. A shorter, harder brush creates a better result. The tip of the brush should be pointy, not round.

#### BEST COLORS

**Fair skin and blondes:** Dark grays and browns are great. All cool tones work well, too. Metallic silver and gold look amazing!

**Medium skin:** Soft bronze pencil liner looks really good. Darker greens, eggplant, and purple work as well.

**Dark skin:** Bright blues and turquoises look amazing! Gold and bronze also work well.

## EYE SHADOW

The palette of eye shadows runs from matte to shimmer, from cool and warm tones to metallic. Women with fair skin can use the lighter color palette; those with medium and dark skin can use darker, brighter tones without looking overdone. Many women agree that eye shadow is probably the most challenging makeup application, right after liquid eyeliner. Start with baby steps, and little by little, after you are more experienced with applying it, you can start using more shadow and really play with the makeup! It's so much fun!

Examine your eyes carefully before applying eye shadow. Feel your brow bone, your eyebrows, the corners of your eyes, and your eyelids and discover their shapes. This will make putting on eye makeup easier. Eye shadow is available in powder, cream, cream-powder, gel, mousse, and pencil formats.

**Powder shadows** offer many looks, from the most natural matte to more dramatic metallic shimmers. They come in pressed and loose formats. The loose ones are often shimmery. Use two brushes for application: no. 1 and no. 2.

**Cream shadows** are very handy and are water-resistant. You can apply them with your fingertips. They are really good in summer, on vacations, and for anyone who lives in high humidity all year round.

**Mousse shadows** are water-resistant and easy to apply: just use your fingers, and that's it. Their texture is whipped and light—great for a quick summer makeup!

**Powder-cream shadows** are usually water-resistant.

**Gel-based shadows** are great for shiny lids. You can use them alone or over powder. They're great for evening makeup—or that '90s heroin look.

**Pencil shadows** are very handy and are usually shimmery. They're a great choice for teenagers or anyone else who is just stepping into the world of makeup, because their application is so easy and fast! They're also great for a quick summer makeup or vacation application.

## CHOOSING SHADOW

Alana is wearing a cream eye shadow in icy blue. Cream and mousse shadows are

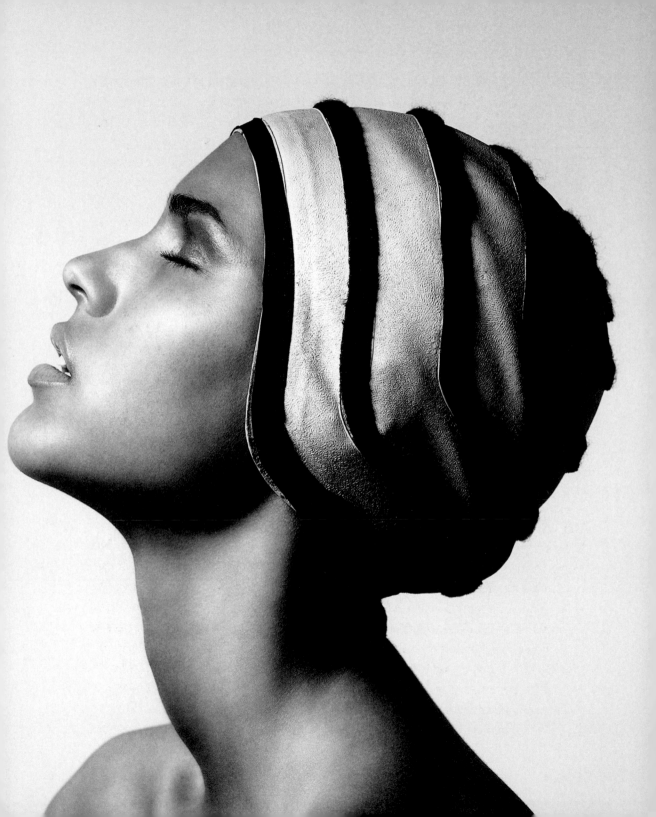

also water-resistant, so if you want to look glam in the water, this is your choice to keep your eye makeup from running (along with water-resistant mascara).

How many times have you bought a powder-format eye shadow because you like the color, but when you got home and tried it on your eyes, there was something that didn't quite work: the color pigmentation was too low, it was hard to get any color on the lids, or the shadow looked matte in the container but after application turned out to be too shimmery or otherwise wrong?

Test eye shadow before you buy, just as you would a foundation. The quality of the shadow is as important as the color.

Test shadow on your hands and ask a makeup artist to demonstrate it so you can see and feel how the shadow works for you.

---

*TIP If you have a problem keeping your shadow on your lids, use a lid primer/eye shadow base product that stops your eye makeup from running. This is especially good for those 40 and up, as well as for those of you who have oily lids.*

*Try your favorite colors first, but be open. You might be surprised to find totally new colors that suit you perfectly!*

---

## HOW TO CHOOSE EYE SHADOW COLOR

If you are not sure what eye shadow to choose, start with a compact of two to five very basic colors: ivory, nude, light brown, medium brown, deep brown, and light gray. Another choice is pastels. They are really light and comfortable to play with, and the result is always natural. Try a combination of matte and shimmer shadows so you can see how the light-reflecting shimmers work on the lids as opposed to the matte ones.

You can choose the colors by coordinating them with your daily wardrobe tones, but it's not a rule at all. Wearing green doesn't mean you would automatically use a green shadow. Yes, it looks good, but you can look just as fabulous with red lips and black mascara.

If you are wearing black from head to toe, black eyes look great and are safe, but how about green? Or mauve? Or keep your eyes open using just matte ivory shadow, and paint your lips fuchsia.

### Small Eyes

Use a shimmer to match your skin color on the inner corners of the eyes. This will give the illusion of bigger eyes. White and metallic liners also give more light on the lids. Use a pencil shadow; it's easier to apply on smaller eyes. Keep your brows clean, because sometimes you can really open your eyes by plucking some hair from your brows and/or making the arch a little bit higher. See an esthetician for that.

### Downward (shape of the eyes)

Keep the volume on the upper lids. Keep the bottom lash line totally clean so it doesn't pick up any "weight." Open the eyes with an ivory matte eye shadow that you apply on the lids up to the crease. Blend well. Use a liquid liner and make wings that go upward, giving your eyes a lift. Curl your lashes and apply black mascara only to the upper lashes.

### Eye Color

Basically, all colors look good, depending how you build up your look to work together: lips, eyes, blush, hair color, and outfit.

**Blue eyes:** Use browns, peach, pastels, gold, copper.
**Green eyes:** Use purple, rose, heather, eggplant.
**Brown eyes:** Use blue, turquoise, plum, eggplant.

*TIP Extended eye makeup looks best as an evening look. Try deeper blue, purple, or green, which look great in matte format. White inside liner makes the eyes appear larger.*

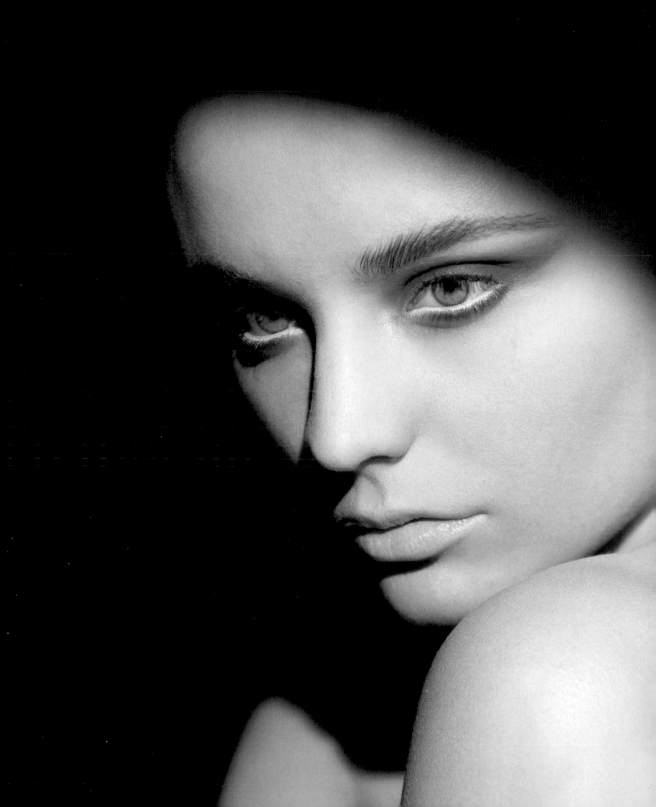

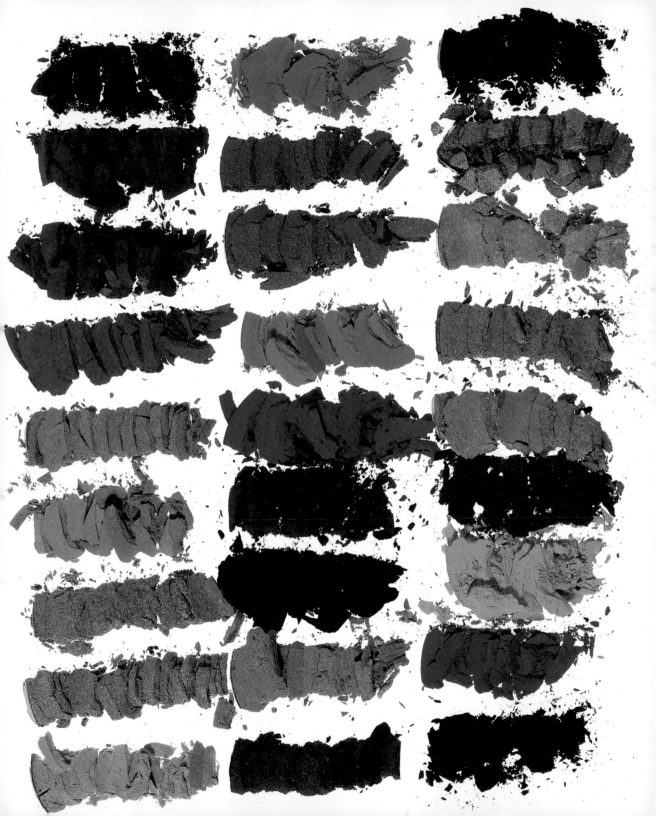

## Hair Color

Hair color is important in making good choices in shadow colors.

**Super/bleached blond:** Cool tones look the best; keep warm tones to lighter shades (light brown, peach, orange, terra-cotta).

**Brunette:** All colors work, especially warm tones. Cool tones can be very surprising, especially dark blues and purples, which really work.

**Red:** The best color choices are green, purple, khaki, and gold.

**Gray:** Warm tones are all beautiful, but deeper purple works as well. An ivory/light gray/black combination is a very classy choice.

---

*TIP* *Make up your eyes first. Apply the foundation and powder to the lids and then follow with the rest of the eye makeup, and wipe the falling powders from your cheeks. The other option is to do the base, as I always do, and tap an extra layer of loose powder onto the cheeks where the falling powders of the eye shadows will land. In the end, you will brush off all the powders from your cheeks. Remember this especially when using darker eye shadows, as well as shimmery and metallic ones.*
*Note: Browns that have too much red will make your eyes look teary and sore.*

---

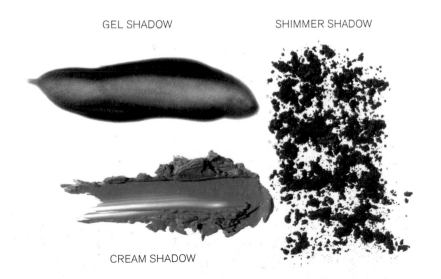

GEL SHADOW

SHIMMER SHADOW

CREAM SHADOW

# Get the Look

**Lydia's flaming red hair was the inspiration for this look which is all about purple matte eye shadow and her amazingly big eyelids.**

*Lydia has perfect porcelain skin, so I needed to use just a very little of a light-formula liquid foundation all over her face, including the eyelids. Then I applied powder.*

*I applied matte purple shadow to the upper lash line and continued to the outer corners and the crease, blending well.*

*I used a smaller brush to apply the same color to the lower lash line.*

*I applied a light gold shimmer shadow to the lids and the inner corners to make Lydia's eyes appear even bigger. I like to use cool tones and warm tones mixed together.*

*I applied black mascara and individual medium-sized fake lashes.*

*I applied a white inside liner to open the eyes and make them bigger.*

*I tapped the cool-tone lipstick straight from the container to Lydia's lips and used the lip liner to even out the color. This gave her lips a softer look, because her eyes are already strong.*

*I applied just a hint of blush color.*

*I finished the makeup with brows (sometimes I do the brows at the end, because that way I can see if I need to darken or fill them at all; in this case I just brushed the brows and set them with a brow gel).*

PHOTO: YU TSAI/MODEL: LYDIA HEARST/HAIR: LOUISE MOON/STYLING: MARTINA NILSSON/NAILS: LIBBIE SIMPKINS

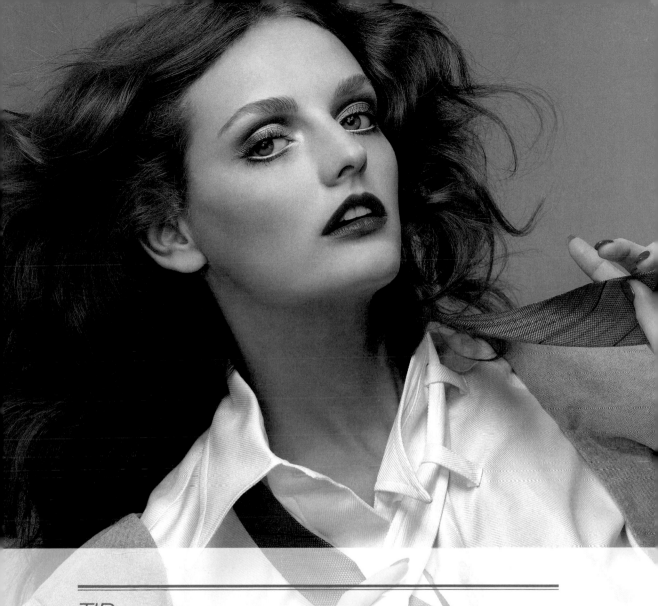

TIP *Before you add individual lashes, apply two coats of black mascara (and maybe a lash primer). When you use a fake lash strip, don't curl your lashes before you add the strip (unless your lashes are superstraight). Glue the strip to the lash line and use a curler to combine your own lashes with the fake ones. Use the curler very light-handed, only to interconnect the lashes to the fake ones—the result looks more natural.*

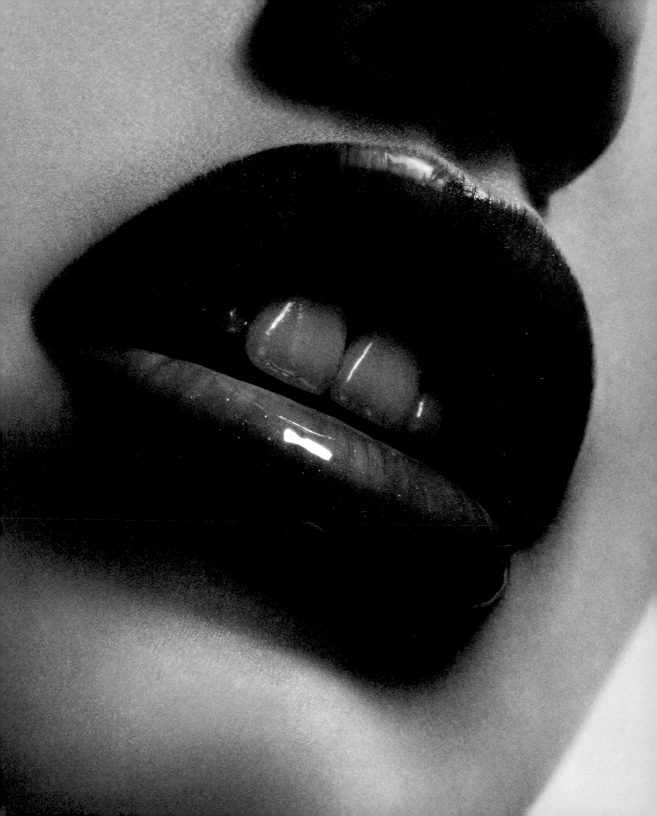

# 15 LIPS

**Lipstick is the most popular makeup item in the world—no wonder, because it is the easiest and fastest way to glam up your face. The history of lipstick is long, all the way from the days of Cleopatra (when lip makeup was made of a mixture of brownish red pigment and scented ointment) to ancient Greece (where women used red lip makeup along with other products). Today's selection is the best ever because of the huge color range, and if you can't find your favorite, you can always make your own color by mixing two or three lipsticks together.**

Use a lip brush or concealer brush for the application, depending on the lip makeup formula and the result you want. A lip brush gives a more defined result, whereas tapping the lipstick on with a concealer brush gives a more relaxed, natural result. I also use my finger to tap the lipstick on the lips. This gives a very natural result as well.

## TYPES OF LIP MAKEUP

**Tinted lip balm:** Gives the most natural result. It is applied directly from the container. This is great for dry winter lips.

**Lip gloss:** Gives instant shine and glam to your lips. Color choices run from clear to black. It's applied to bare lips or on top of already applied lip makeup (lip liner alone or lip liner plus lipstick combination). Application is from the tube with its own applicator or a lip brush.

**Sheer lipstick:** Gives a very natural, moist result. It's a great choice for everyday use. No lip liner is needed. To apply, tap on with a lip concealer brush or your finger.

**Semimatte lipstick:** Gives more coverage as it has more color pigments than sheer lipstick. Lip liner is optional. Apply with a lip brush or concealer brush.

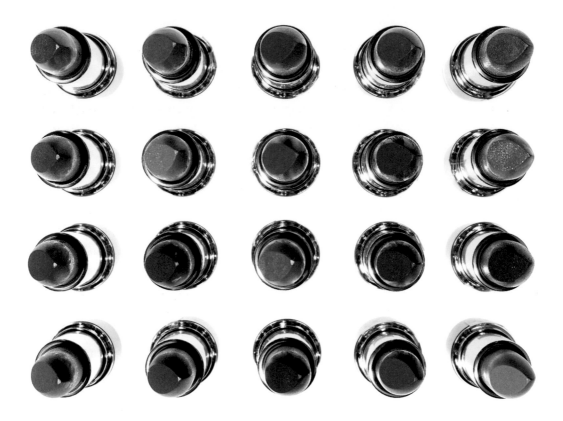

**Cream lipstick:** The color pigments are tight and give you full coverage but still a beautiful smooth, satiny feel. Lip liner is needed. Apply with a lip brush.

**Matte lipstick:** Gives the most coverage. Lip liner is needed. Apply with a lip brush.

**Lip stain:** Gives a long-lasting result but might dry the lips. Apply with a lip brush.

### How do I know what lip color and formula are best for me?

Let's start with the season. If it's summer, you might want a lighter formula, so sheer lipsticks and glosses are excellent choices because you don't want to look too made up under bright sunlight. For autumn you can choose darker shades or keep the lips nude (see chapter 24, p. 164)

Winter is the trickiest because the lips crack so easily, and that is the number one challenge. See chapter 30, "Winter Makeup and Skin Care." I recommend a

STILL LIFE: KIINO VILLAND

tinted lip balm or a creamier lipstick for winter. In the spring, when the sun starts to dominate us, it's time to choose a lighter formula.

If you exercise or you want your lip makeup to stay on longer than normal, use lip stain. The only problem with stains is that they do dry your lips, so I would not recommend using them in the winter or when you feel your lips are dry already. Lip stain is great for holidays, when you want to use lip makeup and don't want to worry about it fading away.

Lip pencils are my favorite. I love the fact that I can use them partially, just lining the lips, and then apply the lipstick or do the whole lip by using a single pencil.

Lip color is a very personal choice. Some days you like nude; some mornings you feel like icy pink, dark burgundy, or fuchsia. Or you want black lips. Or just a clear gloss.

Don't stick with one lipstick or gloss, even if you love the color and the formula; get two to five different colors from the same brand. Using a new lipstick color is a very uplifting experience!

There are also lip pencil lipsticks that provide a look that is always natural: soft and sheer.

Multipurpose sticks that you can use on cheeks and lips are also great, especially on vacation, when you want to pack light. The result is sheer and beautiful.

## POPULAR COLOR CHOICES FOR YOUR SKIN COLOR

**Fair:** Light nude, icy pink, pastels, light peach, fuchsia, bright red, orange red, coral

**Medium:** Medium nude, brown, metallic brown, all metallics, pink, all cool-tone reds; bright corals also look good

**Dark:** Deeper brown, all metallics (bronze and gold mixes), pink, deeper peach tones, bright fuchsia, all reds (if your skin has a more golden-yellow tone, try to avoid orange reds), deeper wine reds; deep eggplant and purple are also excellent choices on dark skin

## LIP GLOSS

Basic lip gloss is a liquid formula and has less staying power than its sister, lipstick, which is wax-based. Try a creamier lip gloss, which tends to stay on a bit longer. Either way you will have to keep reapplying the gloss to your lips during the day. The thicker formula, "vinyl" gloss, stays on a little longer and calls for lip liner. Use a lip pencil before adding the vinyl gloss.

Add lip gloss to the center of your lips and tap it on with a synthetic brush from the center to the corners of the lips. Tapping the gloss will give you the most natural result for daytime. For the evening you can add a little more gloss, but be careful. Never use too much gloss on your lips, because it will start to look corny.

### *How can I create a classy red lip makeup that will stay on through my event?*

Start by exfoliating your lips. Remove all dead skin from your lips to give them a smoother surface.

Then it's time for lip balm. You need to let it absorb into your skin, so wait at least five minutes before you apply the base.

Lip primers are really great if you have lines around your lips. The primer helps prevent feathering and provides a smooth base for any lip makeup product. Just tap the primer onto the lips. Follow with the rest of the makeup.

If you use lip primer, you will have a double "wall" to prevent the color from feathering. After you have applied the foundation to your face (as well as the eyelids), apply loose powder. I like to use a clean eye shadow brush and tap the powder very lightly over the lips instead of using a puff. If you press the powder onto the foundation, you might get too much powder over the lip area, and if your lips are at all dry, they will dry out even more. So be light-handed.

Liquid foundations are the best bases for long-lasting lip makeup.

## LIP LINER

Make sure that your liner is as close as possible to the color of your lipstick. You may have heard that the lip liner should be one to two shades darker, but it looks too '90s to line the lips darker. I also don't like to overline lips with darker liners because they start to look unnatural. A small corrected line will make a difference. Line your lips, fill your lips with the liner, and add a natural brown/nude/light pink-brown color lipstick. Applying a gloss on top will make your lips look bigger.

Make sure your lip liner is neither too hard nor too soft, which will create too-smooth, uneven lines and might break easily. The perfect liner is one that glides perfectly onto your lips thanks to the silicone that is mixed with the waxes. A too-waxy lip liner will hold the lipstick really well, but it also dries out the lips.

Use a sharpener before you line your lips, because you want the point of the pencil to be clean and sharp (I always smudge the point lightly on my hand to round it a little to make application easier).

There is no rule as to where to start lining your lips, as long as the result looks even. I start lining in the middle of the upper lip and go down to the corners to make sure they look even. If not, it's easy to correct the lines with the lip liner pencil. If you make a mistake, use a lip remover swab, wipe the line off, reapply primer/foundation and powder, and start all over again.

After the lines are done, start "coloring" the lips with the liner. You can add a little bit of lip balm at the center of your lips to enhance the pencil's glide on the lips. Color the lips, and after that it's easy to see if there is anything you need to correct before you add the lipstick. Choose a creamier formula that has more color pigment than a regular or sheer lipstick. This is also the secret of long-lasting lip makeup. Many formulas also contain hydrating ingredients, such as vitamin E and avocado and jojoba oils.

Use a lip brush for the application. I always take a small amount of lipstick out of the case, so as not to waste it, and warm it in the palm of my hand before I add it to the lips. Again, there are no rules as to where you should start the application. I start in the middle of the lips, just as with the lip lining. There are several techniques for applying the lipstick, but tapping on top of the lip liner is my favorite, because you will get a really beautiful canvas. For this technique you will need a flat lip brush or smaller-size concealer brush. After the application, press your lips together softly so the lipstick settles down.

Now take a tissue and press it gently to your lips. Tap on a second layer of lipstick. This technique will ensure that your lip makeup will stay longer than normal. If you want extra-long-lasting lip makeup, powder the lips after blotting them. Using a powder brush, tap powder very carefully and light-handedly onto the lips. Then

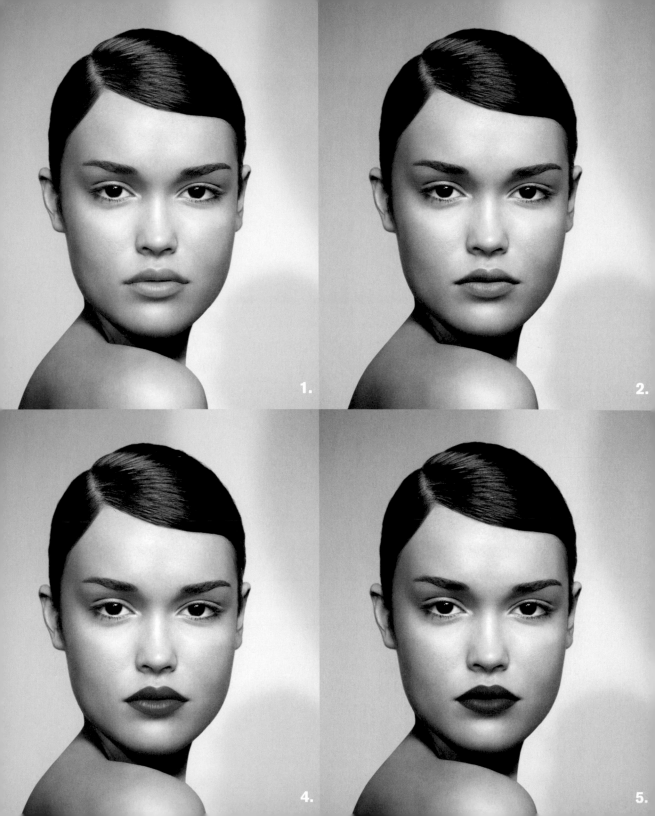

1.

2.

4.

5.

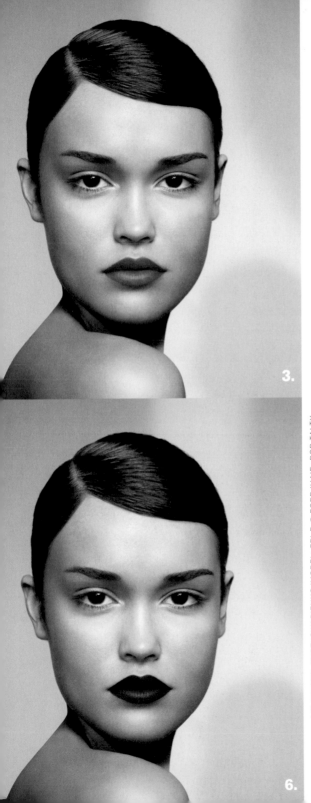

3.

6.

**Changing your lipstick color will
dramatically change your look:**

1. Nude
2. Fuchsia
3. Bright coral orange
4. Aniline
5. True red
6. Burgundy

apply the lipstick by tapping it on once again. This will ensure that your lip makeup is long-lasting! I use this technique in chapter 35, "Cocktail-Hour Makeup."

### How can I make my lips look fuller?

Use a light lip gloss color, which will give your lips a 3-D effect, making them look fuller. You can also use a natural-color lip liner to extend the line to the corners of your lips (be careful not to line over your natural line). Then choose a lipstick close to the color of the liner and finish with a light lip gloss on top. There are also lip glosses and lipsticks that give an instant plump and might last up to five hours. I don't promise you any miracles, but you might see a slightly fuller upper lip.

Darker-shade lipsticks make your lips look smaller, but that can look really cool. Tap semimatte deep red lipstick on your lips, keep your eye makeup light using black mascara, and add some blush for a really great look. Forget routines, myths, and clichés. Try new things. Don't flatten anymore.

### How do lip plumpers work?

My favorite lip plumper is TaberCo's Naked Kiss, which was the first lip-plumping product on the U.S. market, around ten years ago. Now there are many others. Their common ingredient is a vitamin B6 derivative that encourages increased blood circulation in the whole lip area and causes a tingling sensation (you really feel it working!). The results vary. For some they work like a charm; others see few effects.

### My lips are very full. How can I make them look smaller?

Avoid bright colors or glosses. Keep the lips very natural and semimatte. All nude colors are a good choice. Put the emphasis on the eyes.

### Why do my lips get dry?

Lips don't have sweat and sebaceous glands and oils to keep the skin smooth and regulate temperature. Also, the layers of skin on your lips are very thin compared to your facial skin. (More about this in chapter 30, "Winter Makeup and Skin Care.")

### My lipstick bleeds into the small lines around my lips—help!

Try using a lip primer and line your lips carefully before adding lipstick.

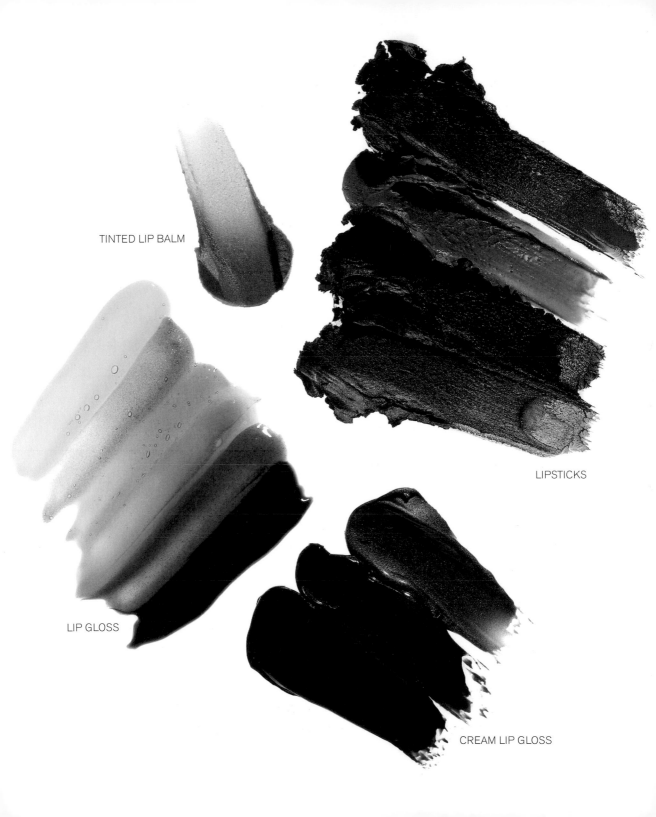

TINTED LIP BALM

LIPSTICKS

LIP GLOSS

CREAM LIP GLOSS

# *No-no's*

**1.** *Dry, chapped lips with matte lipstick. The remedy: exfoliate your lips before applying makeup. Use a tinted lip balm or moisturizing sheer lipstick until your lips are back to normal.*

**2.** *Dark lip liner and drawing beyond the natural lip line. This technique works on drag queens like Lady Bunny, not women.*

**3.** *Too much gloss. The lips end up looking as if they were swimming in a glycerin ocean. A small amount goes a long way.*

**4.** *Half-eaten-away lipstick. The remedy: always carry lip makeup tools with you (lip balm, liner, lipstick, and a brush) to avoid this "look." Always check out your lips after lunch and dinner, before a meeting, and so on.*

**5.** *50+: too-girly lip makeup (too pink). Keep the look classy and elegant. Stick with natural browns, natural light salmon pinks (except for candy pink!), peach, and classy reds. A hint of gloss always looks fresh and gives the lips a beautiful sheen.*

**6.** *Bright lilac lipstick. It doesn't look good on anyone. In fashion shows for fall-winter collections, yes, but in real life it looks scary. Deep purple is a better choice.*

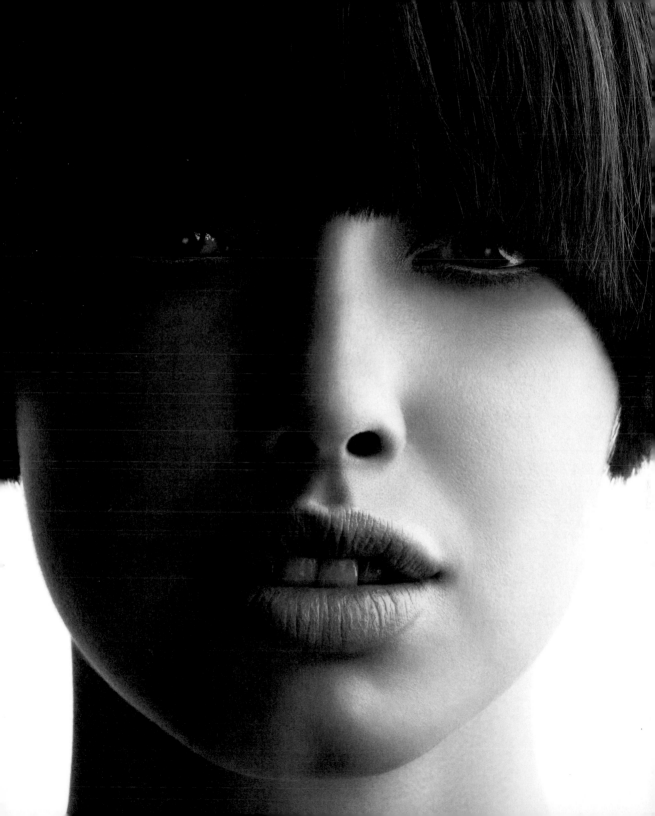

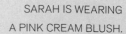

SARAH IS WEARING
A PINK CREAM BLUSH.

# 16 BLUSHES AND BRONZERS

**Blushes and bronzers give the face warmth and life. Bronzers create a natural warmth on your face.**

## POWDER BLUSH

Powder is the most popular and the easiest blush to apply, and it comes in an extensive variety of colors. Powder blush is applied on top of powder foundation so it glides beautifully onto the base. Powder format is for everybody, but it's an especially good choice for oily skin, and also for skin with enlarged pores. That's because powder keeps the skin looking matte longer.

## CREAM BLUSH

Cream blush is a great choice if your skin is very dry or you are 50+ (the skin is drier and has deeper lines, so cream blush looks more natural on the skin than powder does). Use it on top of the foundation; no powdering needed. If the result is too shiny or too bright, you can fade it by powdering the blush area lightly. If you want a dewy result, you can mix the cream blush with a day cream or tinted moisturizer in the palm of your hand and apply it to the face—a very natural result!

Cream blush leaves the skin with a beautiful, healthy glow and is also an excellent choice for summer or nightclub makeup, when you want your makeup to last in the humidity.

PHOTO: KURT ISWARIENKO/MODEL: SARAH @ _A MODELS/HAIR: LOUISE MOON

## GEL BLUSH

Gel blush is the most unpopular format in today's makeup world, but it was widely used in the 1920s, when the flappers went for that round dot of rouge on their cheeks. Gel blush gives a very natural, sheer result but might start looking quite dry after a while, especially if you have dry skin. It is a great choice if you play sports, though, because it dries on the skin and has staying power.

### Where should I apply blush?

This is the question I've been asked the most. I always ask my clients to look into a hand mirror and smile. The blush should go on the apples of your cheeks, on the outer side of the iris. Don't use the blush on your forehead or nose or under your chin. That was done in the late '70s and in the fashion editorials. Keep your look natural. That's state of the art.

### What is the right technique to apply the blush?

Apply powder blush with a brush; cream and gel blush should be applied with your fingers, a foundation brush, or a sponge.

Start on the apples of your cheeks and slide the brush toward the hairline with small twirling motions. Use the same technique with cream and gel or liquid blushes, when you are using your fingers. Tap the product on the cheeks with a sponge and then blend it with the clean side of the sponge. A foundation brush is also good for cream blush, but we professionals love to use our fingers for cream formats because you really feel the product and can warm it up between your fingertips and welcome it to the skin.

### What blush color will suit me?

Fair skin: light icy pinks, corals-peaches, tawny; olive-asian skin: brighter pinks (too icy looks too ashy) and browns-coppers; dark skin: reds (including bright fuchsia), wines, and oranges. The more color you have, the deeper or brighter blush color you need. Red hair looks amazing with peach tones, which keep the whole look safe and natural, but pinks also look good.

Choose your blush color to coordinate with your eye and lip makeup. Then everything will come together. Sometimes you can apply the blush first and follow with the eye makeup. Maybe you will add less as a result? The order of application makes you see your makeup in a different light! So try a different order.

### Should I get matte or shimmer format?

Matte is more practical because it looks the most natural. Shimmers are fine, but I would leave them for evening looks. Those 40+ should always use a matte formulation.

### How should I choose a bronzer?

Your skin tone is the most important factor when choosing a bronzer. If you are fair, you want to stick with light sand and gold bronzers to make your face look sun-kissed but still natural. If you have slightly tanned fair skin, it's okay to use deeper colors like terra-cotta and deeper sand colors. Those with a medium to

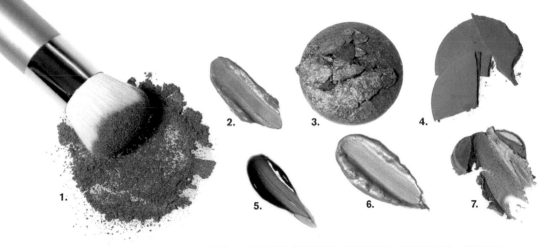

**VARIOUS BRONZER FORMULATIONS: 1.** LOOSE POWDER FORMULA, WHICH IS APPLIED WITH A VERY LARGE POWDER BRUSH ALL OVER THE FACE OR LOCALLY ON THE APPLES, FOREHEAD, NOSE, AND DÉCOLLETÉ. BE LIGHT-HANDED! **2.** BRONZE MOISTURIZERS GIVE MORE COVERAGE. **3** AND **4.** PRESSED POWDER, WHICH IS THE EASIEST TO APPLY. **5.** GEL BRONZERS ARE GREAT AND GIVE A SHEER RESULT BUT DON'T COVER ALMOST ANYTHING. **6.** CREAM FORMULA IS GOOD, BUT YOU SHOULD ADD A VERY LITTLE AT A TIME. **7.** STICK (HERE A GOLDEN STICK THAT LOOKS GOOD ON VERY LIGHT SKIN).

Mediterranean skin tone can use deeper bronzer colors, and dark skins look fantastic with gold and bronze mixed bronzers because the light reflection looks very natural on darker skin. If fair skin is tanned, those work as well.

## HOW TO CHOOSE A BRONZER

Just as with blush, choose a matte type for daytime. For evening, shimmer bronzers look terrific.

Powder or cream bronzer? Pressed powder bronzers are the handiest, fastest, and easiest to apply and are great for everyday city-life use. Apply on the apples of the cheeks with a blush brush to give the most natural result.

A cream bronzer is great in the summer because it takes humidity well. Use it on top of your base (tinted moisturizer works really well), no powdering. Apply with a foundation brush, a sponge, or your fingers. If your skin is oily, skip the cream bronzers and stick with powder (when the skin exudes too much oil, the cream bronzer will slip off). Gel bronzers are the sheerest and don't cover; they just give a healthy glow. I like bronzers in a stick format, as well the cream blushes. They're very handy and easy to apply.

# *No-no's*

1. *Dark bronzer on a pale face, especially in the middle of winter. I don't necessarily like bronzers in the winter at all. Use them during later spring and summer, when the natural sunlight gives your face a beautiful light.*

2. *Sparkly and shimmery bronzer during the daytime. 40+ women: don't use shimmery bronzers at all. Matte looks more sophisticated and makes the skin look younger.*

3. *Orange bronzer, especially matte orange.*

4. *Bronzers on the eyelids.*

STILL LIFE: KIINO VILLAND

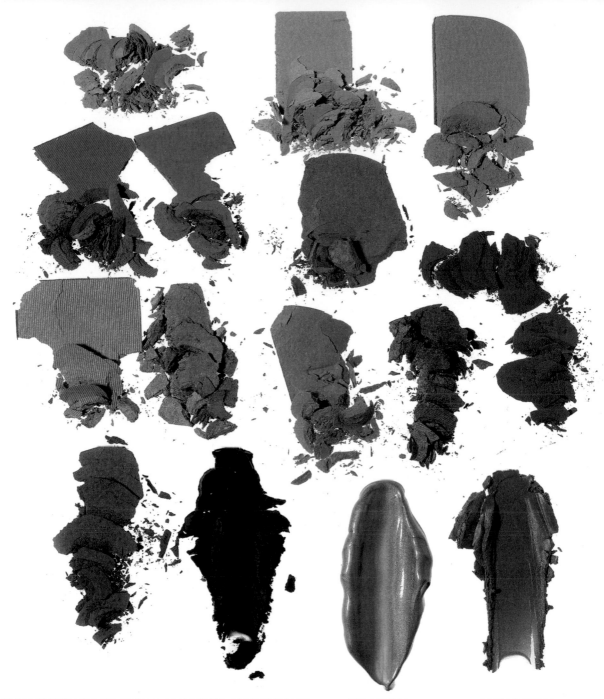

GEL BLUSH                    CREAM BLUSH

THE POWDER FORMULATION IS THE EASIEST AND FASTEST TO
APPLY. THEY COME IN EVERY COLOR AND TONE YOU DESIRE AND
ARE A MUST FOR OILY SKIN TYPES. CREAM BLUSH IS A GREAT
CHOICE IF YOU HAVE DRY SKIN OR YOU ARE A 50+ BEAUTY.

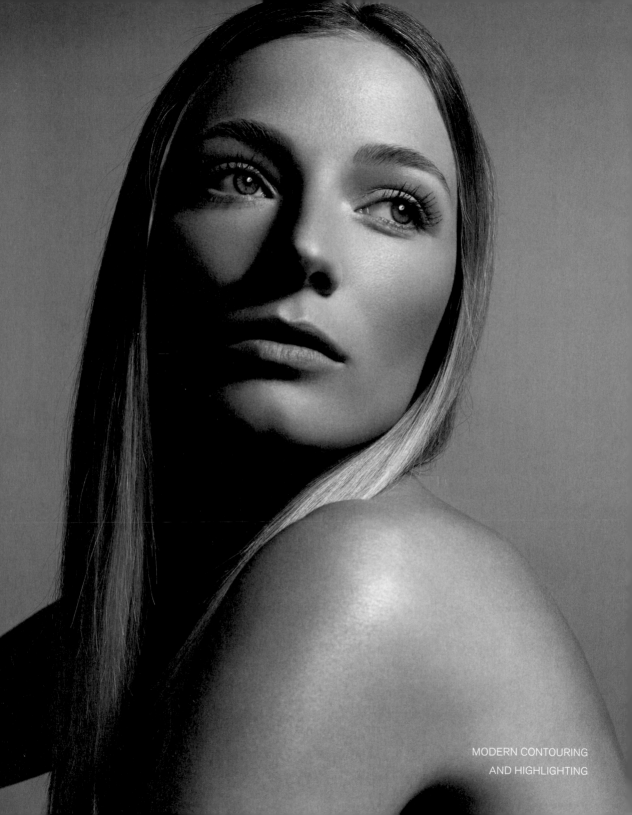

MODERN CONTOURING

AND HIGHLIGHTING

# 17 CONTOURING AND HIGHLIGHTING

PHOTO: PASCAL DEMEESTER/MODEL: ANA @ LA MODELS /HAIR: KEIKO HAMAGUCHI

**Contouring is a very basic makeup trick and has a long history, but it can be very confusing. It's very old school to use it all over your face. The old-school goal was to give the face the "perfect" oval shape look, making the nose look shorter or thinner, adding a product under the chin to "lose" five pounds, or minimizing forehead. This works for stage makeup. But it's far from natural in daylight, even when it's done with a light hand. Contouring your whole face will actually change your face into somebody else's and make you into a character. I am against your trying to "change" your face from round or square to oval shape, which is way too old-fashioned for today's modern women. You'll look your best working with what you've got.**

Modern contouring gives you natural shades for your cheeks. Suck your cheeks in and apply matte bronzer in the hollows. Blend well; otherwise it will look like it's been done for a Broadway performance. Contouring the eye creases will make your eyes appear larger. Forget about contouring the nose, chin, and forehead. That never works in real life, in raw daylight.

**There is no ideal shape for a face. You are most beautiful with your own face shape.**

Highlighting is the modern way to bring out your cheeks and give the face extra light and lift. Know where to apply the product on your face. I like to use highlighting on the eyes, cheeks, bridge of the nose, and chin. But remember that a very little goes a long way! Too much highlighting makes you look like a walking full moon, and highlighting works the best on summer makeup, as well as on evening makeup, because the face really comes alive when the light hits it.

Use the darker shade of your eye shadow duo in the crease of your eyes to make your eyes bigger, and the lighter shade in the crease to open up the eyes.

If you have small eyes, adding a small amount of light shimmery eye shadow on the inside corners really opens up the eyes. When the light hits the shimmer, it gives the illusion of more space between the eyes. (See chapter 25, "Shimmer Makeup."). Matte, darker blush terra-cotta, dark tile, or bronze colors, for example, work well to emphasize your bone structure.

Highlighting accentuates the areas in your face that naturally have a light-reflecting or 3-D effect: the cheekbones, forehead, chin, and bridge of the nose. I like shimmer highlight powder for that use because it stays on the best. Always use the powder format on top of base (tinted moisturizer or liquid foundation plus powder), never on bare skin, because it won't stay. Powdering is important because no powder-format makeup product will slide beautifully and easily if you don't use powder first.

Use your blush brush to apply the shimmer to the face. I always swirl the product in the palm of my hand with my brush before applying. Apply a bit to the highest area of your cheeks to bring out the cheeks, or you can highlight the whole T-area for an evening look. Highlight your face after you have done the rest of your makeup, so that you'll really see what you're looking for. You might need only a simple cheekbone highlighting. Another possibility is a cream highlight product, which often comes in a handy, easy-to-apply stick. Cream highlight is for you if your skin is dry or you're in a hot climate. It's also an excellent choice for more mature skin, especially for

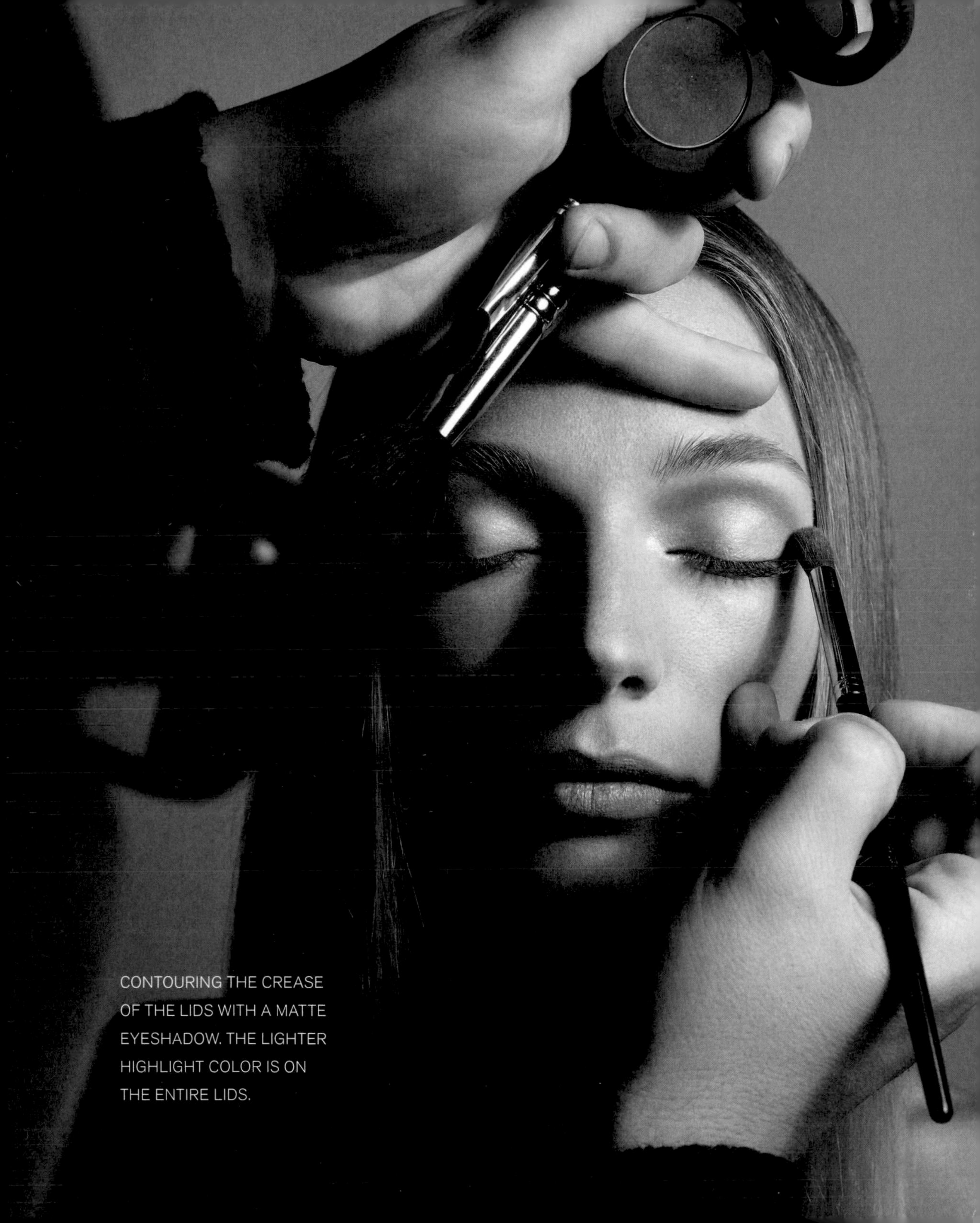

CONTOURING THE CREASE
OF THE LIDS WITH A MATTE
EYESHADOW. THE LIGHTER
HIGHLIGHT COLOR IS ON
THE ENTIRE LIDS.

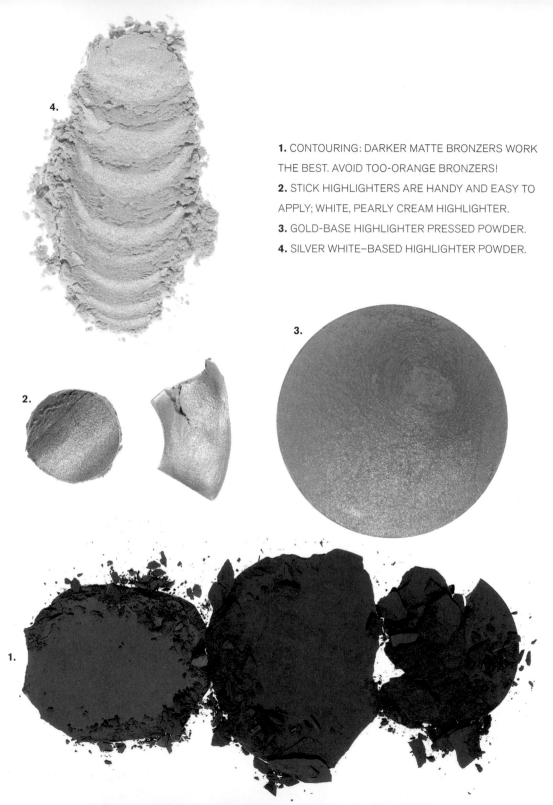

**1.** CONTOURING: DARKER MATTE BRONZERS WORK THE BEST. AVOID TOO-ORANGE BRONZERS!

**2.** STICK HIGHLIGHTERS ARE HANDY AND EASY TO APPLY; WHITE, PEARLY CREAM HIGHLIGHTER.

**3.** GOLD-BASE HIGHLIGHTER PRESSED POWDER.

**4.** SILVER WHITE–BASED HIGHLIGHTER POWDER.

summertime evening makeup. A hint of cream highlight on your cheeks really brightens the face and gives you a fresh look. Add cream highlight on top of your foundation. Don't powder, because then you dry out the skin and make the shimmer look matte.

Use your fingertips, a foundation brush, or a sponge to apply cream highlighter. Test which ones you like the best. And remember to blend well!

Highlighter pencils are also very modern and superhandy; they are available in liquid pencil and cream pencil formats. You can highlight your eyelids and cheeks in just a minute! Blend well with your fingertips.

Liquid highlighter is a little trickier, but I use it by mixing it with a liquid foundation and applying it directly to the area where I want it to stay. If it is not mixed with the foundation, it looks too obvious and won't blend into the skin naturally and beautifully. We professionals use this technique quite often, but for your everyday use I would suggest the powder and cream-stick formats—easier and faster!

You can also highlight your whole body for an evening red-carpet look; more about that in chapter 43, "Body Makeup," with supermodel Alessandra Ambrosio.

# No-no's

*Don't use too much highlighting in your makeup if your skin is oily or superdry or you have enlarged pores. Oily skin is shiny anyway, so there is no point in adding extra shine to your skin. A matte look always looks better on oily skin. Any highlighter product on very dry skin makes it appear even drier and flaky. If you have enlarged pores, forget highlighter products as they will make your pores very noticeable.*

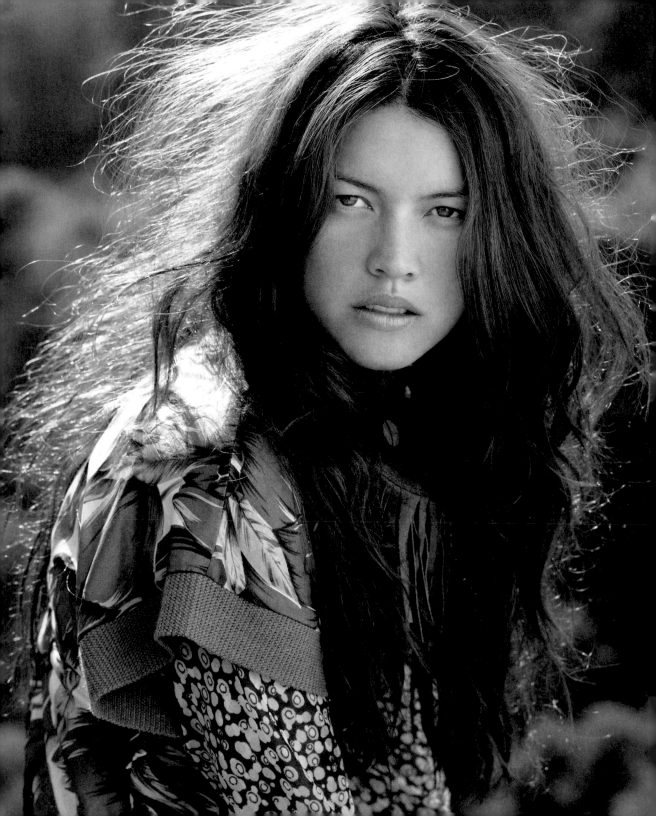

PHOTO: KURT ISWARIENKO/MODEL: A_ENE/HAIR: DAVID VON CANNON/STYLING: TIM BITICI/PUBLISHED AT THE A-MAGAZINE ITALY

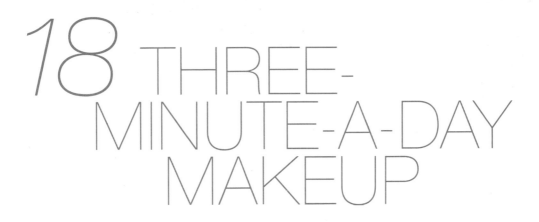

# 18 THREE-MINUTE-A-DAY MAKEUP

**Women don't have a lot of time to spend on their makeup. The most important consideration is your outfit. For example, you don't need to wear nude makeup if you wear nude clothes. Here are some ideas to prepare yourself for a busy morning.**

## THE PREPARATION

Make sure that your eyebrows are well groomed.

If your lashes are superstraight, get an eyelash perm, so you don't have to spend time curling your lashes.

Make sure you use the skin care routine appropriate to your own skin type.

## THE PRODUCTS AND TECHNIQUES

**Tinted Moisturizer** with SPF 15 to 20. There are oil-free to more nourishing ones, so make sure you choose the right one. If you have oily skin, apply a mattifier primer to keep the makeup on your face longer. If you have dry skin, apply daily moisturizer before tinted moisturizer. Apply a small amount all over the face, including the eyelids. This will even out your skin, and it looks the most natural and radiant.

**Loose Powder:** Apply lightly all over your face to keep your makeup from running.

**Black mascara:** Apply one or two coats to your upper lashes.

**Blush:** Try a warm peach.

**Lipstick:** Try a natural pink lipstick tapped onto the lips with a synthetic brush.

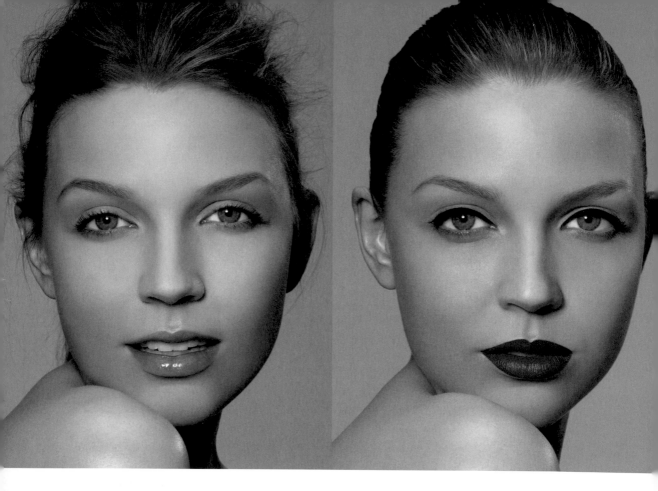

# 19 A.M. TO P.M.

You have five minutes to do your makeup in the morning and will celebrate your first anniversary with your husband this evening. He is taking you to a very nice restaurant for dinner. You need to prepare in the office in fifteen minutes.

## THE PREPARATION

**7:15 A.M.:** After showering, apply your daily moisturizer and eye-area cream and have breakfast while the creams absorb into your skin before you apply makeup.

## THE PRODUCTS AND TECHNIQUES

**8:00 A.M.:** Add tinted moisturizer with SPF 15 to 20. After you apply tinted moisturizer, use concealer if needed, especially at the corners of the eyes. Powder your face. Use black mascara, peach color lip gloss, and a peach blush, all warm tones, clean and fresh. Splash on your eau de parfum, and voilà! At 8:15 A.M. you're on your way!

**5:00 P.M.:** Check out your base and correct it with powder to give a beautiful semimatte finish, great for an evening look. Apply the product on your eyelids as well as the top of the lips.

Apply liner to the middle of the eyes and draw the line to the outer corners. Finish the lines to draw the eyeliner to the inside corners as well. Make the lines thinner toward the inside corners.

Brush your eyebrows, but don't fill them and make them too "perfect" because the look is already glam; keep it modern. Line your lips carefully with red lip liner and fill the lips with the liner by coloring them. This makes your lips matte, and you won't need a separate lipstick at all! Now brush your hair and make it modern and classy!

**5:20 P.M.:** You catch a taxi, and Mrs. Anniversary is on her way!

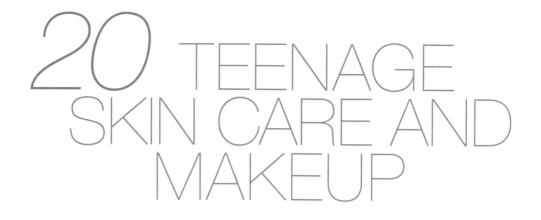

# 20 TEENAGE SKIN CARE AND MAKEUP

The day you start to use makeup, you must also start to use skin care products. Clean makeup off your face with a cleanser or cleansing wipes and then moisturize your skin. That's it; it takes two minutes. And don't forget to use a sunblock SPF 15 to 30, especially in the summer. If you live where there is sunshine all year round, sunblock lotion is your number one day cream. For combination and oily skin types, always use oil-free products that don't clog the pores. If you have a blemish, use a blemish-control gel at night to dry it out.

## MAKEUP

There is no specific age when you should start using makeup, but I would say that fifteen is a good age to start experimenting. You should take baby steps: black mascara and clear or light pink or peach lip gloss are enough to begin with.

I know that all your idols (singers, actors, etc.) may wear a lot of makeup and you might think it looks cool, but the fact is that it's made for photo shoots, the red carpet, and TV. It won't look that cool in real life. Less is more!

You really don't need any foundation. But if you want something to cover up, you should use a concealer that blends into the skin (see page 81).

Use concealer only to cover the redness of a pimple. You can't make it disappear completely.

Blush will make you look too made up.

Eye makeup should be light. You can use matte or shimmer formulas.

All cool eye shadow tones work very well on all skin tones.

For very pale to fair skin tones, pastels are a great choice; for medium to deeper skin tones, purple, bright pink, and fuchsia, as well as blue and turquoise, are excellent choices.

For eye shadow or eye pencil, just apply the product on the lash line and blend it a little to soften the line. If you want to make your eyes pop more, apply a bit of color on the outer corners of the bottom lash line.

Don't pluck your eyebrows too early. Natural brows are great and beautiful.

Manicures are fun to have with your friends. You can play with all the rainbow colors you want; use your imagination and have fun! Airbrushed nails are also very popular; you can get any theme you want: a leopard pattern, a little heart, polka dots—you name it!

You should not start pedicures at an early age. I would say to wait until at least age sixteen.

Just have fun in your youth, and don't take makeup too seriously.

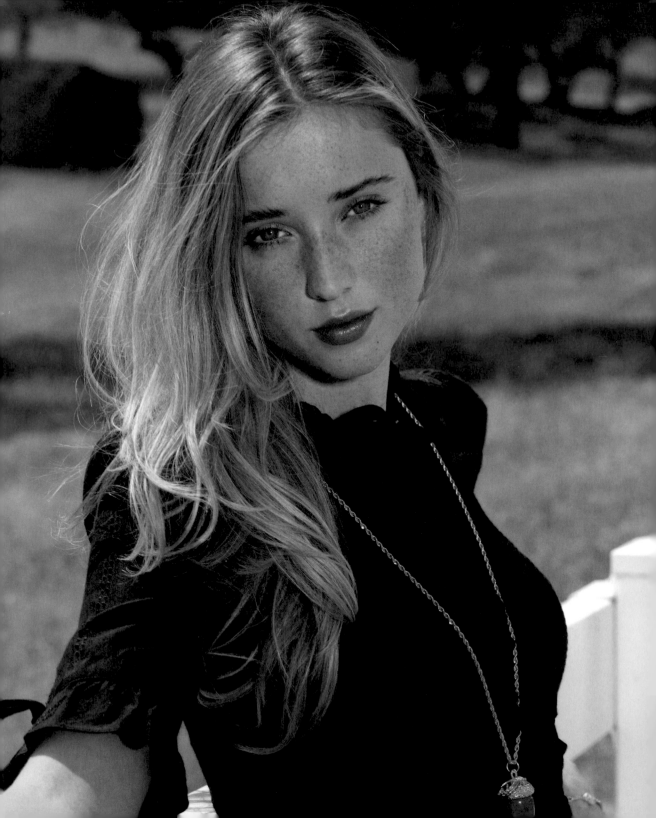

# Get the look

*Here's the five-minutes daytime look for 17-year-old Amanda.*

*She is wearing SPF 30 sunblock to protect her skin from UV rays.*

*I applied black mascara on her upper and lower lashes and then combed it through with a lash comb.*

*Then I applied light pink lip gloss.*

*I finished the look with a touch of pink blush. I applied it right on her cheekbones to create a natural look.*

## Ole Henriksen on Teen Skin Care

*Clean skin is the foundation for healthy skin, so you are never too young to start using a gentle foaming face cleanser. All parents should introduce their children, both boys and girls, to a ritual of washing their faces every morning and night. This ritual should start at age seven. Moisturizer is equally important for boys and girls. Sun protection is a must, even for babies. A regular moisturizer, used daily, should become the norm from age 14 and ideally contain SPF 15. A light-textured moisturizer is best suited to young skin, since the skin at that age is well hydrated.*

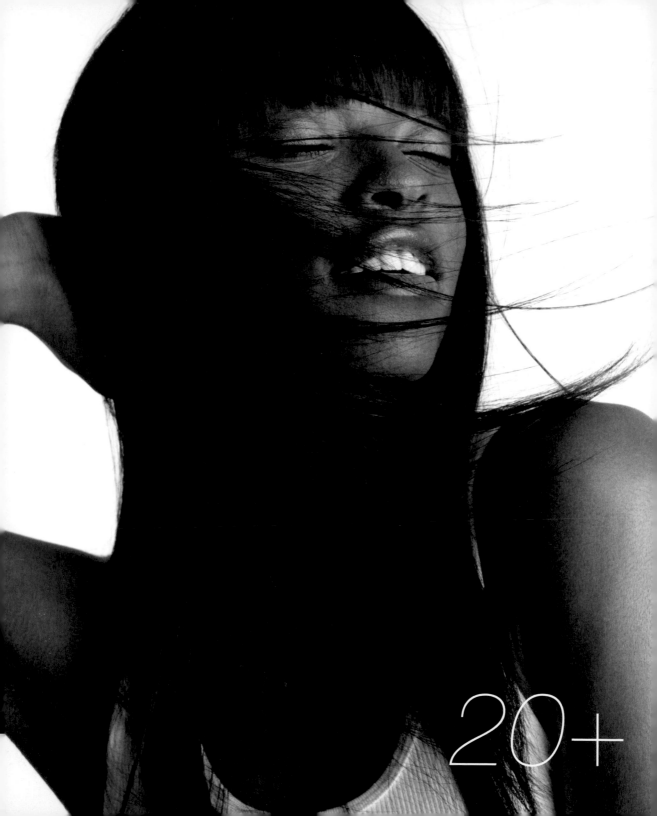

20+

# 21 BEAUTIFUL AGE

PHOTOS 150–157: PASCAL DEMEESTER/MODEL: ANNECA/HAIR: KEIKO HAMAGUCHI/STYLING: HEIDI MEEK

**Every decade of your life is an award you've received, and you should carry yourself with your head high. All ages are gracious, and even as you get older and notice the changes on your face and body, you should remember that aging is a natural process and it's not the end of the world. Making the right choices in diet and exercise, getting enough rest and sleep, following the right skin care routine, and having a good haircut/ color and makeup make a great difference. Makeup has an amazing uplifting effect that can really create a beautiful appearance, whatever your age. I talked with six beautiful women, all different ages, and asked them questions about their personal skin and makeup routines. All the makeup I suggest is for everyday use and doesn't take more than fifteen minutes. One thing that unites these ladies is they all love makeup!**

## 20+ BEAUTY

Anneca is a 20+ student, full of life and energy. With her outgoing personality, she is not afraid to try new makeup colors, and she loved the cool-tone eye makeup I used. 20+ makeup should be fun and daring, because this is when you can really play with bold colors and shimmers without looking too made up.

But how about skin care? Sometimes young women forget the importance of skin care. When you're young, you don't really think about it. But when you hit 30 you wake up and realize that you should probably have worn that sunscreen after all! Start good skin care practices before the damage is done.

Sometimes 20+ skin might still be fighting acne, so you must see a dermatologist to develop the best skin care program, designed just for you. A good 20+ skin care routine is cleansing, toning, moisturizing, and protecting. You should also start using eye-area creams or gels at 20+.

Once a week, exfoliate (if you have oily skin, do this four times a week, or you can exfoliate every day with a mild exfoliating cleansing cream) and use a face mask after the scrub.

For oily skin, use a clay mask four times a week. If your skin is combination, use a clay mask locally on the oily areas of your face. For dry skin, use a deep hydration mask.

## TIPS

- *Tinted moisturizer is the best. Don't use a heavy base.*
- *If you have blemishes, you can cover them using a little concealer. But don't use too much concealer on top of a pimple: the more you use, the more it will stand out.*
- *Differentiate between day and night makeup. Glitters don't look good in daylight.*

## 30+ Beauty

Heidi is a fashion stylist and has a very busy lifestyle with meetings and running around to catch the latest trends. Sporty, natural Heidi doesn't wear much makeup, and she describes herself as more of a tomboy than a fashionista.

At 30+ there are more photodamages to the skin, and some fine wrinkles. You should start using lift serums and firming night creams along with your daily skin care routine. And don't forget the eye-area cream or gel.

If possible, see an esthetician for a facial once a month to keep your skin and pores clean.

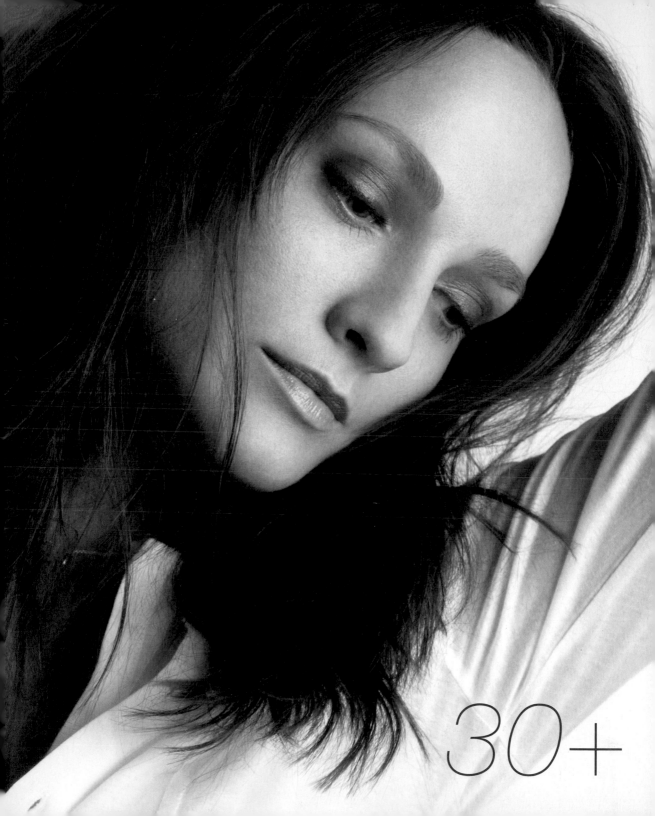

30+

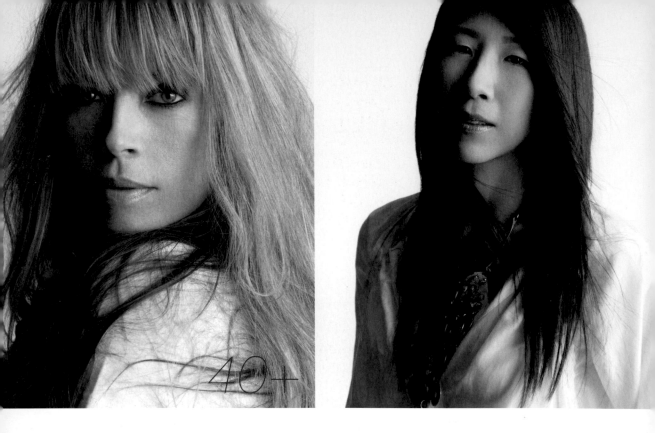

## 40+ Beauty

Business manager Shell is a good example of a 40+ woman who mixes her cool looks with the business world. This businesswoman doesn't have to wear the most conservative makeup—no way! Today's businesswomen are individuals.

Creative director Ann has one of the most beautiful complexions I have ever seen, thanks to her Asian genes and her healthy diet, which keep her skin firm and luminous.

## *Ole Henriksen's Tips*

*Invest in a peeling system for home care. Use it twice a month. Many home care kits incorporate the benefits of both a microdermabrasion and an acid peel and may include a mask as well. Simultaneously, I would cut out all sunbathing on the face by always covering the face when sunning the body. On a daily basis, use a firming collagen-strengthening serum prior to the application of a day cream. Purchase a richly textured eye cream containing peptides for added firming benefits. For night care, I suggest the layering of pigment-fading and cell-renewing serum, followed by the application of a cream of a variety of natural acids that will stimulate the skin's cell turnover rate. Within a week, your skin will begin to look more radiant and youthful, with a soft, smooth texture and better tone and resiliency.*

## 50+ Beauty

When I first met Kristin, I noticed her positive energy and her heavenly laugh, which filled the makeup room. Happiness and joy are beautiful. Smiling is beauty.

# Ole Henriksen

*With each passing decade, the skin becomes drier, especially when going from 40+ to 50+. At the same time, the collagen in the dermis layer has become less soluble, which manifests itself in more obvious expression lines and some lost skin elasticity. The need to use richer-textured creams and switch permanently to a lotion cleanser based on a high concentration of essential fatty acids is the main difference between treating skin that is 40+ versus 50+.*

*Brown spots on the skin are hyperpigmentation, caused by excessive production of melanin, by pigment cells (melanocytes) that are present in the epidermis just below the stratum corneum, the skin's top layer. The main culprits that cause brown spots to appear are extreme sun exposure, various kinds of medication, hormonal changes in connection with pregnancy, and birth control pills. Dermatologists typically prescribe products containing hydroquinone to make the melanocytes dormant. Hydroquinone is outlawed in most countries outside the United States, and rightfully so, as the strong and toxic chemical may fade the hyperpigmentation fast but the slightest amount of sun exposure, even when using SPF, will make the discoloration come back tenfold. I like to*

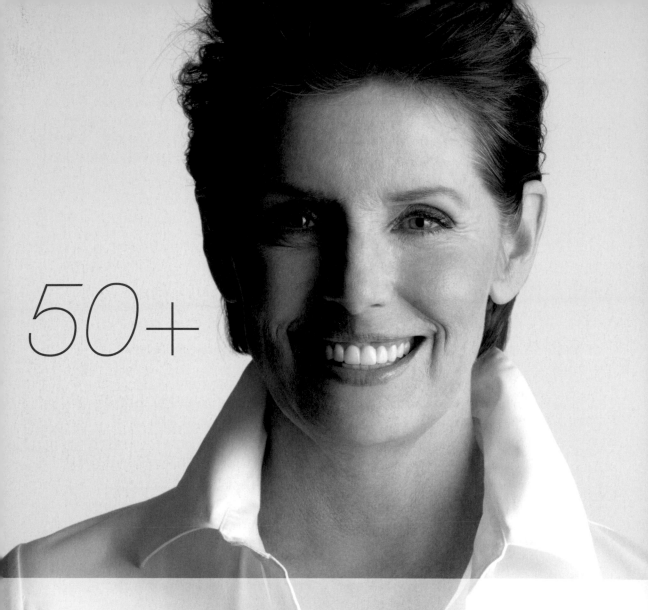

50+

*lighten spots with natural extracts. It takes longer, but the result will last. The natural ingredients are lactid acid, mulberry extract, licorice extract, lemon extract, sugar maple extract, sugarcane extract, and a new extract called Actiwhite, from peas and sucrose. Using a 2.5% concentration of Actiwhite over a six-week period has effects similar to those of hydroquinone, but without causing sensitivity or irritation to the skin.*

**70+ BEAUTY**

Marlene is an amazingly classy lady. She takes the best care of herself with her skin care routine, and she loves makeup, especially dark red lips!

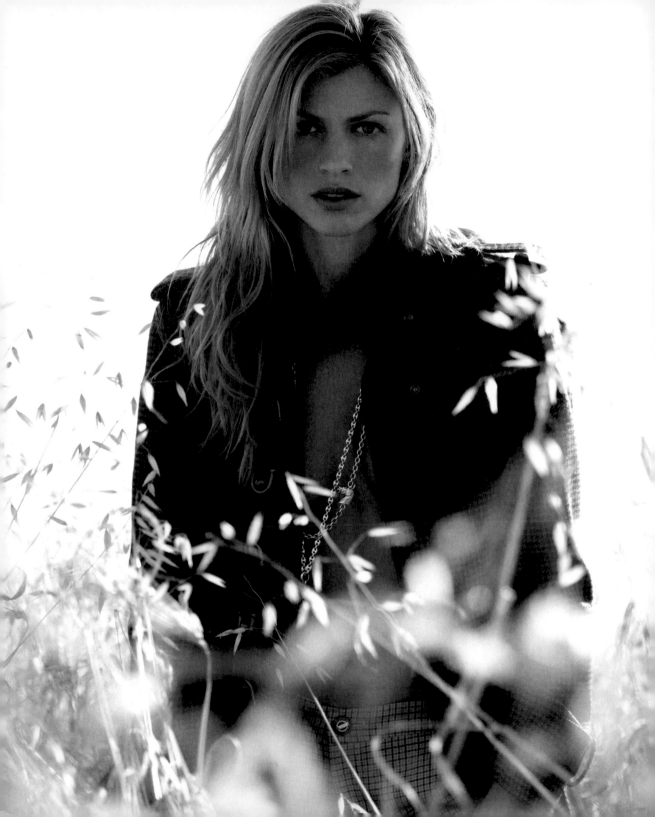

PHOTO: YU TSAI/MODEL: DANIELA URZI/HAIR: BERTRAND W./STYLING PETRA FLANNERY/PUBLISHED AT HARPER'S BAZAAR INTL.

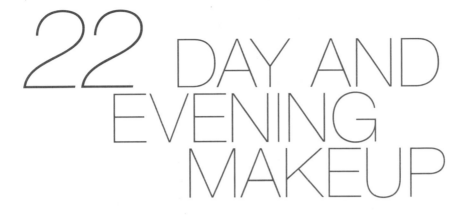

# 22 DAY AND EVENING MAKEUP

**Natural matte colors work well for professional looks or for an important job interview when you want to look like your natural self but still be well put together. Matte makeup is also an integral part of an oily skin makeup routine.**

## Get the Look: Day

*A serum, daytime moisturizer, eye-area cream, and lip balm were applied to Daniela's skin. For oily skin a mattifying primer is a must, for shine-free skin and longer-lasting makeup.*

*I then applied tinted moisturizer with a foundation brush and a triangle-shaped makeup sponge, remembering the lips and eyelids.*

*I then applied loose powder to make the skin matte, a must for this look. (Keep a compact powder with you. If you have oily skin, use oil-blotting papers.)*

*I then used a light sand-color matte eye shadow that is close to Daniela's skin tone to keep the eyes really neutral, applying it on the lids up to the crease. If you have oily lids, use a special eye primer for eye makeup. It keeps the eye shadow and liner in place.*

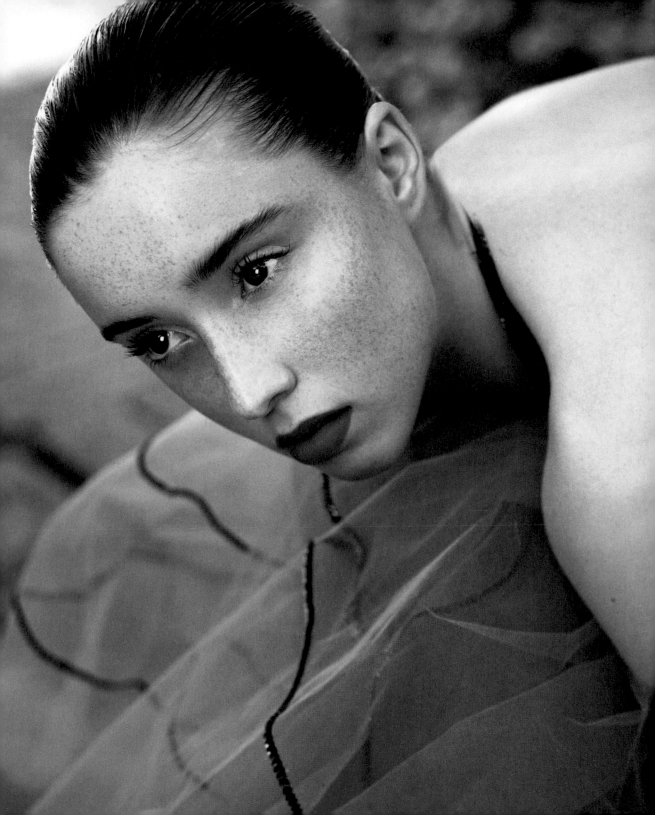

I then applied a coat of brown-black mascara. I used a heating eyelash curler after applying the mascara. This is really easy for those of you who are not familiar or comfortable with a regular lash curler.

---

*TIP* If your skin is combination, use more powder on the T-zone than on the rest of the face, which is drier. By pressing the powder puff firmly to the skin, you ensure that the powder will set on the foundation. Repeat twice on the oily areas of your skin. At the end of the application, use a big powder brush to take any extra powder off your skin.

---

I then groomed her eyebrows using a brush to direct the brow gel to keep them in place. The lipstick is a matte natural shade applied with a flat lip brush. The blush is a warm peach color on the apples of Daniela's cheeks. The result is a beautiful and practical daytime look.

# Get the Look: Evening

A serum and a moisturizer were applied to Amanda's skin, as for day makeup. If you have oily skin, use a mattifying primer.

I then applied a very sheer tinted moisturizer, to keep the skin looking natural, and loose powder.

I left the eye makeup very natural, using just light brown eye shadow and black mascara.

I brushed Amanda's brows straight up and placed them with a hairspray (I sprayed a strong-hold hairspray on the eyebrow brush and brushed the brows upward). This makes the makeup look fresh and young.

I lined Amanda's lips and applied the same color of cream matte lipstick.

# 23 DEWY MAKEUP

**Dewy makeup gives the skin a healthy glow that is not overly shiny.**

## Get the Look

*I massaged YaYa's face with a moisturizer to give a good base for this look. Then it was time for the tinted moisturizer, the secret to this dewy look. I used a very small amount to get the most natural result, applying it smoothly all over the face with a foundation brush, and doing the eyelids and lips as well. I finished by tapping the tinted moisturizer into the skin with a sponge.*

*I powdered only the eyelids and lips.*

*I chose the lightest pink shimmer eye shadow, which I applied all over the lids, and used black mascara on only the upper lashes.*

*Finally, I applied light pink shiny lipstick by tapping it on with my fingers, plus light pink blush to finish the look.*

*YaYa's brows were naturally beautiful, so I just brushed them and used a little bit of brow gel to keep them in place.*

*Her white manicure looks really cool and fresh.*

PHOTO: YU TSAI/MODEL: YA YA/ONE MODEL MGMT/STYLE: MARTINA NILSSON/NAILS: JENNA HIPP

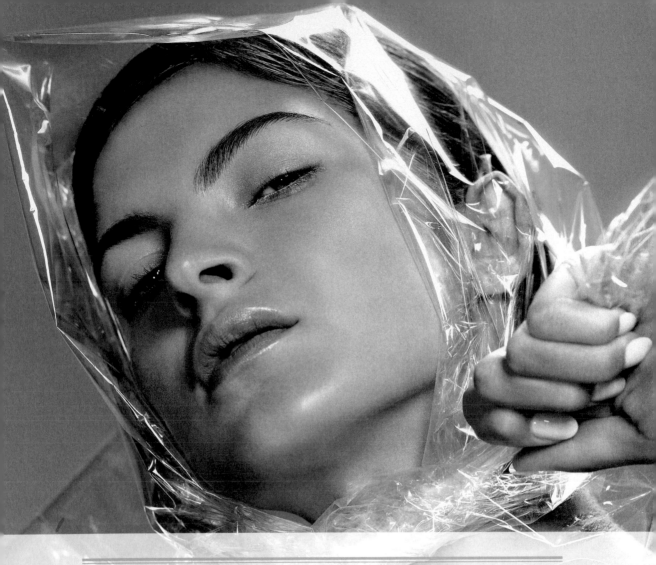

*TIP* *Dewy makeup works best for dry to normal skin or combination skin that is more dry than oily. This is because oily skin exudes too much oil naturally and the skin starts to look too shiny. But if you love this look and your skin is oily, prepare the skin with a clay mask, a mattifier toner, and a stop-shine product before applying the tinted moisturizer to keep the skin matte naturally, but fake it by adding the dewiness with tinted moisturizer. If you need to use a concealer, you can do so after applying the tinted moisturizer, but please blend it in well!*

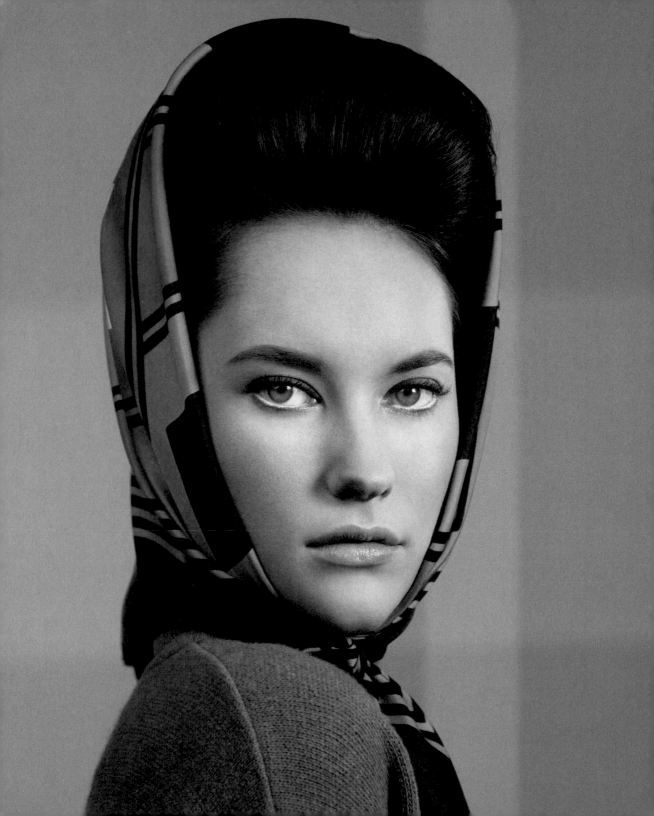

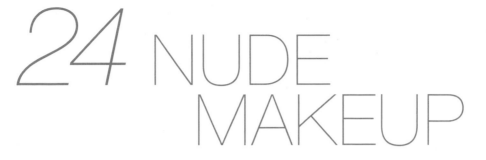

# 24 NUDE MAKEUP

In nude makeup, the colors are washed out and the face looks minimalist. Nude suits all skin tones, from fair to dark. Good advice to remember in doing the nude look is to make the eyes pop a little, because nude lips and totally nude eyes will look ghostlike. The basic nude colors are light brown sand colors, light yellow/orange-based browns, and pink-based light brown mixes. For dark skin tones, keep the lip color to darker brown and brown-pinks, because too-light ones will look washed out and ashy. By using a liquid foundation or concealer on the lips, you can make your own nude lips. Don't powder the lips, because they might get too dry. I like matte or semimatte nude lips, which look more natural than glossy ones.

## NUDE HARMONY

This classy nude makeup is very easy to create because all the color tones blend together easily. This look will work very well as your autumn look, when the leaves are turning brown and orange.

## Get the Look

*I applied a green-toned color corrector primer to balance the redness of the skin.*

*I then applied a light-formula liquid foundation and loose powder to create a perfect matte base. Matte skin looks better on daytime nude makeup. I applied a medium-brown matte eye shadow to the lash line and blended in.*

PHOTO: KURT ISWARIENKO/MODEL: RACHEL @ PHOTOGENICS/I-AIP: KRISTIN HEITKOTTER

Then I used a white matte inside liner to open up Rachel's eyes, to give a hint of modern vibe with the '60s look. I always use white kohl before I apply any other makeup product on the bottom lash line or lashes, because it won't mess up the lashes.

I applied eye shadow on the bottom lash line to create depth.

I used a matte medium-brown eye shadow on the eyebrows also. I filled and brushed them to get a natural but defined result.

I used dark brown-black mascara and curled Rachel's lashes with a heating curler.

I applied nude lipstick, using a lip brush to get a soft look with no hard lines. Sometimes you can do so-called foundation lips, in which you apply liquid foundation to your lips to cover them, giving a totally washed-out look. It works really well if you are wearing black mascara.

I used a soft warm-tone blush; peach works beautifully on this makeup, because it brings warmth to the face. Remember to apply the blush to the apples of the cheeks.

## Get the Look

I used an oil-free moisturizer plus primer top to encourage the makeup to keep from running (when you dance and get sweaty).

I powdered the skin lightly, but I didn't want to make it look as matte as the daytime nude makeup look. Evening makeup looks really good with slight highlights on the lips, eyes, and cheeks. I did the eyes to look more futuristic and to stand out with an ivory semishimmer eye shadow that I applied all over the lid with a bigger eye shadow brush. Matte dark gray eye shadow was applied to the crease to make the eyes look rounder.

I applied black liquid liner on just the roots of the lashes, and used a pair of fake lashes to deepen the look. Clear adhesive is the best.

I applied another very thin line of liner on top of the lash line to make the strip "disappear."

I brushed the eyebrows straight up with the help of a brow gel. This mades the makeup look edgier and cooler.

I applied light pale pink–salmon lipstick with a lip brush.

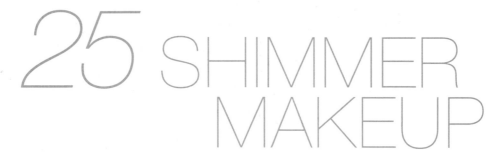

# 25 SHIMMER MAKEUP

**Shimmery makeup is more popular than ever because it gives you instant glamour with a light-reflecting look.**

Shimmer can be found in foundations, powders (both loose and transparent), eye shadows, blushes, lipsticks, pencils, and even mascaras. Shimmer is made of light-reflecting crystals called mica. Use shimmer products anywhere you would use any highlighting cosmetic product, on the areas of your face where the light would reflect naturally: cheekbones, forehead, chin, bridge of the nose, eyelids, lips, décolleté, and all over the body (shimmer body lotions). Shimmers suit all skin colors. On deeper skin tones I love to use metallics (gold, silver, bronze) as well as cooler shades such as purple and ocean blue, and turquoise. Bold shades such as orange, yellow and fuchsia also work beautifully. I love using shimmer products on my clients, but I always use a very small amount. Be careful not to use too much, because you don't want your whole look to be supershiny. Shimmer looks fine in fashion and beauty editorials, but in real life you must be much more light-handed.

## Get the Look

*The shimmer look works beautifully as a day look or natural evening look.
I kept the skin totally matte (this look is great even if you have a drier skin
type or you have impurities, because the shimmer is not in the foundation).
I applied a light brown matte eye shadow in the corners of the eyes with
a small eye shadow brush and followed the natural line of the crease.
I used a bigger brush to blend the eye shadow to create a subtle crease.
I applied white shimmer eye shadow on the middle of the lids, using a small*

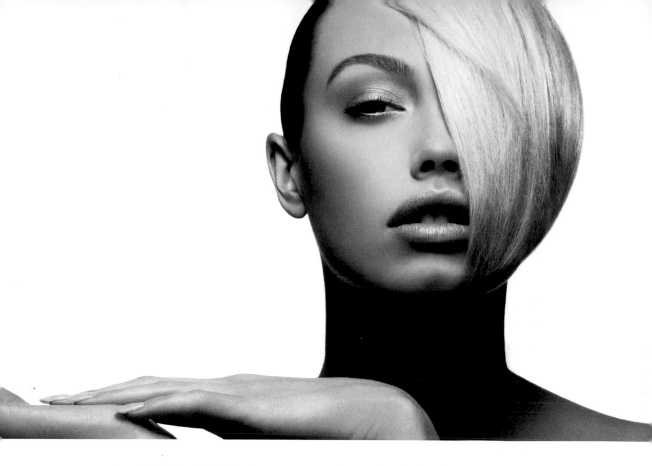

brush to blend it to the inner corners to create a light-reflecting effect.
I curled the lashes and added black mascara.
I applied light, cool-toned shimmer moisturizing lipstick with a lip brush. No lip liners for this look.
I used white inside liner (kohl) to open the eyes and to provide a "wake-up call."
I used matte, deeper pink blush to contour the model's round face.
Shimmers are very popular in spring makeup looks. Shimmer body lotions enhance a great evening look. If you are wearing a dress that shows your legs, body bronzers give you a beautiful sheen, and if you are pale, it almost looks as if you're wearing shimmery stockings.

If you wear a more open dress (showing your arms and décolleté), you can use body bronzer all over your body, but mix it with a moisturizer so that it won't cake on the skin, especially if you have dry skin. Again, a very small amount goes a long way!

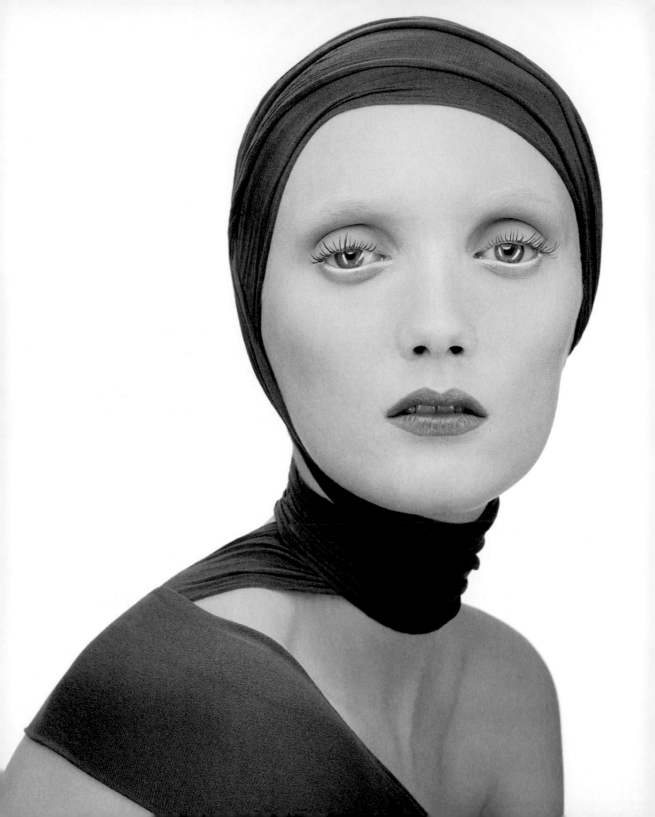

# 26 BOLD COLORS

**Bright, bold makeup colors are always a great choice when you want to lift up your look. Use them as color therapy.**

Play with colors—a bold blue eyeliner or bright coral lips, or both. Remember that nail colors can also be unusual: orange, yellow, blue, green-turquoise. Bright colors look the best in spring and summer, when clothes are colorful. Then your colorful face will blend naturally with a green floral dress or fuchsia chiffon blouse. You can also play with opposing colors, which create very exciting tension: green with red, purple with yellow, and blue with orange.

## Get the Look 1

*Tools: matte green eye shadow, black mascara, individual lashes, matte orange lip liner*

*I made the eyes look rounder, applying the shadow all the way up to the crease and blending it well.*

*I applied black mascara and individual lashes.*

*I curled the natural lashes and the individuals together with a heating curler.*

*The lashes will interconnect, and the result will look very natural.*

*I lined the lips with bright orange-coral liner.*

*I applied peach blush to the temples, just a hint to give the face warmth.*

# Get the Look 2

**Tools:** *blue-turquoise matte eye shadow, black individual lashes, black mascara, peach-orange lip gloss*

*First I bleached Ira's brows to give the eye shadow more room.*

*I used liquid foundation and transparent loose powder for a matte effect.*

*I applied the eye shadow to the roots of the upper lash line and blended it well.*

*I extended the shadow from the outer corners of the eyes outward.*

*I didn't blend too much, and I made sure that the shadow didn't extend all the way to the temples, to avoid the '80s futuristic Nina Hagen look.*

*Add the color also on the bottom lash line: black pencil liner on the lashlines and black kohl inside the rim.*

*Add black mascara and individual fake lashes.*

*Finish with peach gloss.*

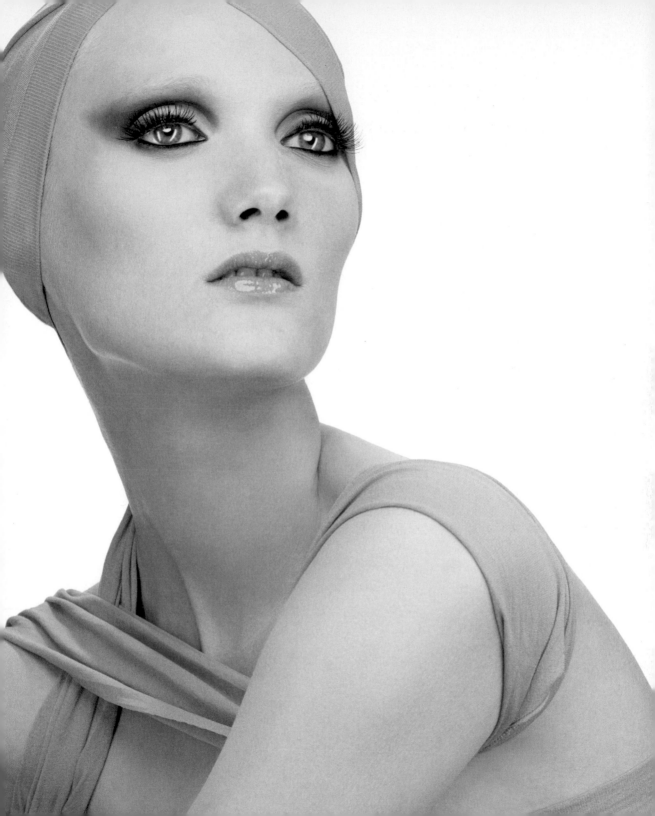

# 27 BLACK MAKEUP

**Black is one of the most-popular and most-sold colors in makeup: mascara, eyeliner, kohl, eye shadow, nail polish, and even lipstick and gloss.**

Black suits everyone, and it's a very easy color to work with, because you see the result on your face immediately. When working with lighter tones such as pastels (or any lighter versions of a color), you might not see color on your face right after the first touch or application. Black doesn't always have to be strong, but I made these two makeups look more fashionable and bold so you can really see what you can do with black. You can see much lighter versions of black on actress Anne Archer in chapter 34, "Modern Evening Makeup."

## EYES

Black eye shadow is great if you blend it well. And by blending and smudging the lids with a kohl pencil you will get perfect, fashionable smoky eyes. You can also create a lighter version with less color and liner, but you must blend and smudge them together well.

# Get the Look

**Tools:** *black matte eye shadow; black kohl; three eye shadow brushes: no.4 for applying the color, no. 6 for smudging and blending the color and kohl together, and no. 5 for applying the shadow to the bottom lash line; a Q-tip for smudging the bottom lash line and fixing any mistakes*

*First I applied tinted moisturizer, plus I made the skin editorial looking by tapping a little bit of Vaseline on Kim's T-zone with my fingers to catch the light.*

*I started with the matte eye shadow, which I applied on Kim's upper lash line and blended with the no. 6 brush, back and forth like a windshield wiper. The black color will fade into the gray, and you might need to add a bit more black eye shadow from time to time during the application to keep the shape and intensity. I used the no. 5 brush to apply the black eye shadow to the bottom lash line and blended it with a Q-tip. I extended the eyes a bit to look more like cat's eyes. When you extend the eyes, be light-handed, so you won't overdo the look to runway makeup (that is absolutely creative and cool-looking too, but doesn't suit for a daytime use) by using the no. 7 brush.*

*I used black kohl on Kim's inner rims as well as on the lids, instead of a black pencil liner. Why? Because kohl is softer; it blends and melts perfectly on top of the eye shadow. I applied the kohl to the roots of her lashes and blended and smudged it with the no. 4 brush to create depth for this look.*

*I crowned the look with two coats of black thickening mascara.*

*I applied clear gloss to keep the face in balance.*

*I didn't use blush, because we have the highlights (and sometimes you can skip the blush, to keep the makeup simpler, especially with these strong makeups).*

*I then applied black nail polish.*

# Get the Look

*Tools: black eyeliner pencil, black matte lipstick, lip brush*
*I applied a light-formula, oil-free liquid foundation. It's important to apply the foundation to the lips as well to get a good, even base so that the black lip makeup will stay well and longer.*

*I powdered the face and lips lightly.*

*There aren't really black lip liners on the market, so I used a black eyeliner pencil (kohl is too soft and the lip lines would have become too smudgy) to line Christine's lips. After lining I applied a black matte lipstick with a lip brush to finish the makeup.*

*I didn't use eye makeup or blush, to keep the rest of the makeup really simple; otherwise it would have gone far. Now it's cool and wearable.*

*Go, girl!*

PHOTO: WARWICK SAINT/MODEL: CHRISTINE /HAIR: GIO CAMPORA/NAILS: LIBBIE SIMPKINS

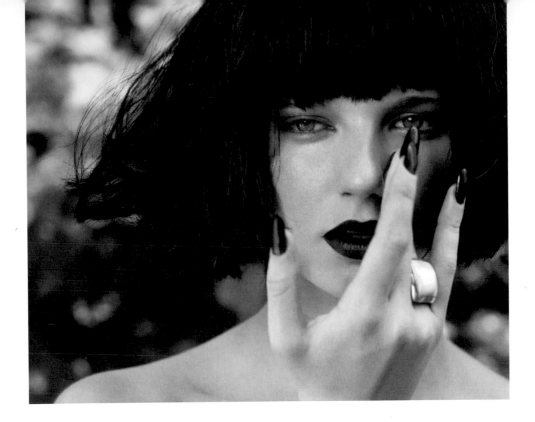

## BLACK ON LIPS

Black lip makeup is not commonly worn in everyday life, but it is a great statement maker. Black lips were extremely popular in the late 1970s and early 1980s, when punk and New Wave in music and fashion were born. The icons were British bands and singers like Toyah, The Cure, and Boy George, who painted their lips black (or rainbow colors). Black lipstick made a return in the mid-1990s with the advent of grunge.

Today black lips are back. The young generation has rediscovered the gothic look (it really never went away, anyway).

Even the most conservative daytime makeup junkies love to project a strong attitude by wearing a black lipstick in the evenings. And why not? Makeup should be full of surprises. I think it's fabulous to do something different and unexpected every now and then. Give yourself a totally new look, and see if your friends (or your husband!) even recognize you.

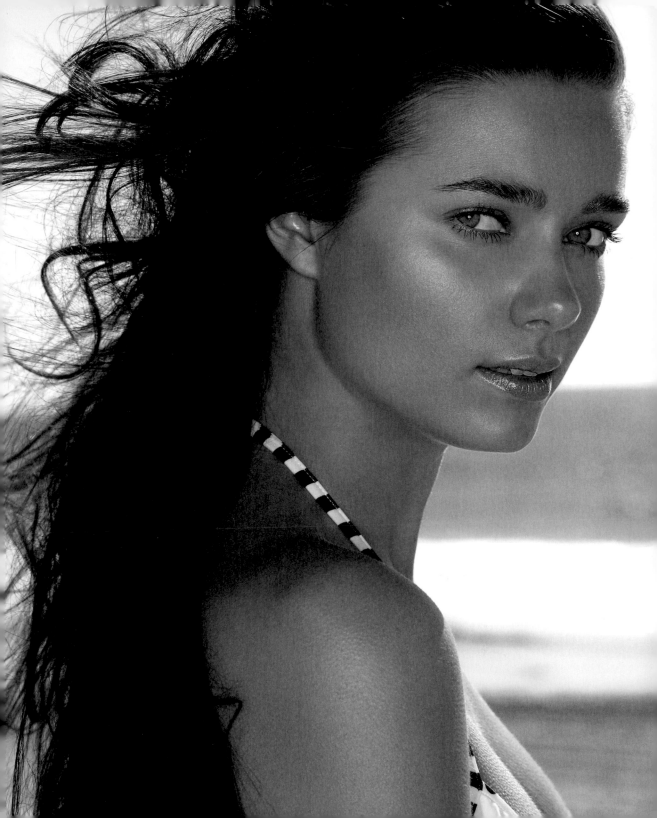

# 28 SUMMER LOOKS

PHOTO: NADIA PANDOLFO/MODEL: ALICIA @ ELITE/PUBLISHED AT FOAM MAGAZINE

**Makeup for a summer day must be easy and fast. No one likes to waste time in front of the mirror when the sun is out! I created three different summer vacation looks: sporty, summer glam, and dusk.**

## Get the Look: Sporty

*This is for those who like to be active on the beach but still want look neat. A sporty summer look takes five minutes or less to do—simple and beautiful.*

*I used an oil-free face and body sunblock with SPF 30 and UVA/UVB protectors*

*I used a water-resistant face and body shimmer on Alana's arms, legs, and décolleté to give a beautiful shimmering effect. I applied the same product to her face, but only on the cheeks, forehead, chin, and nose to deepen her tan, blending well so that the shimmer "melted" naturally into the skin.*

*I used a makeup sponge for the application.*

*I used a creamier face and body shimmer, which is easier to work with than watery/gel-based products, which are good for the body but hard to work with on the face.*

I applied a terra-cotta cream eye shadow on the entire lids, using my fingers.

Black waterproof mascara is a must. You can also try green, blue, or turquoise waterproof mascaras. They look great on summer days!

I applied lip balm with SPF 35 and UVA/UVB, with clear moisturizing gloss on top.

Nails should be natural and short—more practical when playing beach ball, Rollerblading, or surfing!

# Get the Look: Summer Glam

When vacationing in a beautiful resort and wearing a fabulous swimsuit, you should always glam up your face as well. This makeup is not meant to be used for swimming or playing volleyball on the beach but for hanging around the pool and partying, it's more than perfect.

She applied a body sunblock with SPF 30 and UVA/UVB protectors.

I used a special compact foundation with SPF 42 and UVA/UVA protectors, which is a perfect summer makeup base because it protects the skin and makes it look even, especially when you want to look your best at a pool party. Use it all over your face, including the eyelids and lips. I powdered the face (lips and eyelids as well) with a very light hand to give a little bit more matte result. A too-dewy look on fair skin on a bright summer day makes the skin look too oily.

I filled Alana's brows with a dark gray eyebrow pencil to make them look full and arched. Brow pencils are better on summer makeup, because they are wax-based and tolerate humidity and water better than matte eye shadows used on brows.

I used no eye shadow, just black waterproof mascara.

PHOTO: DANIELA FEDERICI/MODEL: ALANA @ ELITE/HAIR: DAMIEN MONZILLO/STYLING: HANI/PUBLISHED AT MADAME, GERMANY

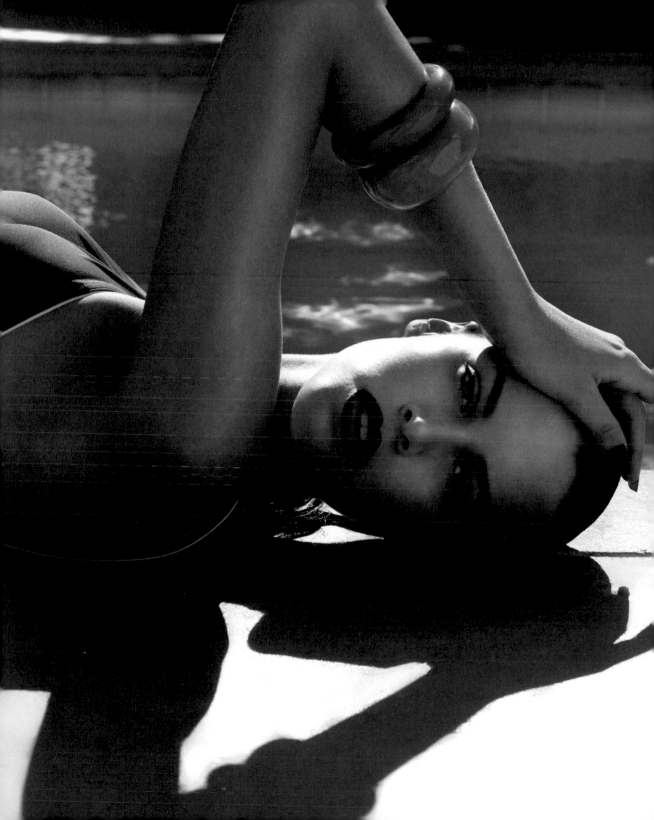

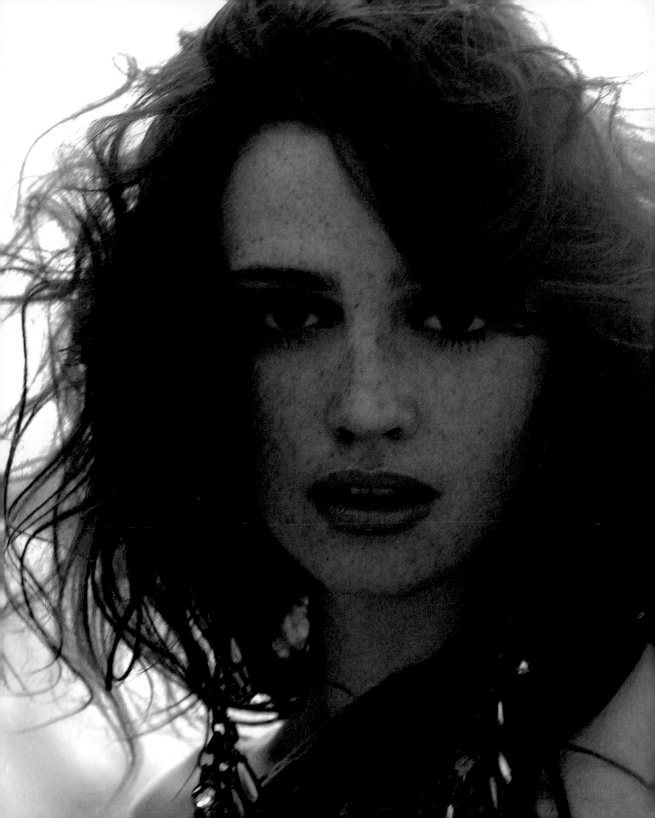

I lined the lips very carefully, filled the lips with liner, and then applied a glittery red lipstick on top of the liner. The glitter sparkles in the sun and makes the makeup more fun, especially when you are vacationing and partying.

Long red nails are elegant and superglamorous and go hand in hand with the lips.

# Get the Look: Dusk

Summer evenings are beautiful, especially at dusk, right before the sun goes down. It's probably the most beautiful light on Earth (at least I think so). In Scandinavia the sun never goes down for two weeks in June, and in California the sunsets are amazingly beautiful. So much inspiration for the makeup! I wanted to use bolder colors on Jodie's face to bring out the summer feel.

I applied a special aloe vera gel for calming and soothing the skin after she spent the entire day in the sun.

I used tinted moisturizer and light-handed powdering.

I chose deep purple for Jodie's eyes and applied it to the entire lids to give more depth.

I used three coats of black mascara to achieve the "spider eye" look. Don't wait for the mascara to dry between applications, because it's too hard to apply second and third coats once it's dry.

Orange lipstick is a summer color for everyone. I didn't line the lips, just used a lip brush. Now it's relaxed and cool.

Make your nail color orange too. It works really well.

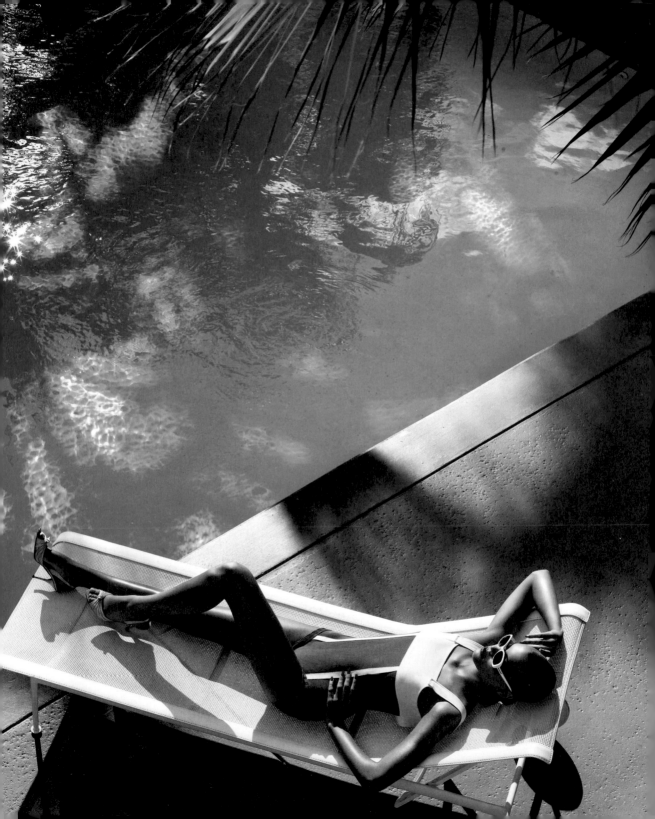

# 29 TANNING

**Until the twentieth century, only poor and working people who spent most of their time outdoors had tanned skin. The upper classes kept themselves as pale as possible even though sunbathing was thought to cure illnesses and prevent diseases. In 1902, a Swiss doctor named Auguste Rollier opened the world's first sun clinic, seating patients outside to expose them to the sun and let them breathe the fresh air of the Swiss Alps to cure various diseases, mostly tuberculosis.**

Everything changed in the mid-1920s, thanks to Coco Chanel, who tanned her skin during a vacation on the French Riviera. Women on both sides of the Atlantic loved her new look and started to copy her. Also, the sensational Josephine Baker's caramel-colored skin had a role in making sunbathing into the new hype!

In the 1940s and '50s tanning was enhanced with baby oil and metallic sun reflectors. In the 1960s, the James Bond babe Ursula Andress showed the world how to look modern in tanned skin and '60s makeup, and the Beach Boys gave the world the tanned surfer look.

In the early 1970s the first tanned Malibu Barbie was born and the new hit TV series *Charlie's Angels* made the California tan look superfashionable. It wasn't until 1978 that the first SPF 15 sunscreen was made for the mass market and understanding the importance of protecting the skin with better products than baby oil started to become more widespread.

In the 1970s and '80s, fashion was all about tanned skin; all the cover girls of the major international fashion magazines were deeply tanned.

The grunge look of the '90s was all about looking pale again. In Asia (Japan, Korea, China, and some parts of India), it's very popular to look pale. It's not surprising that Asians wear wide-brimmed hats and carry parasols and umbrellas to protect their skin from UV rays. And that is smart.

You don't need to lie by the pool for hours to get that sun-kissed look; you can tan yourself with self-tanning lotions or by getting a spray tan in a salon. Both are extremely popular today, and the good thing about them is that they are safer for your skin in the long run than spending time under the sun.

## HOW TO TAN

The image of healthy, tan skin is beautiful. But even if it looks sexy and fashionable, it doesn't suit everyone. If you have fair, Irish-Scandinavian skin, you won't get tanned and it's better for your health not to try. You should avoid the sun and wear SPF 30 throughout the year.

But you can still get a nice tan at a professional tanning salon by having a few mild tanning treatments on a tanning bed or using a spray tan! Medium and darker skin types tan more easily and should use SPF 15 even if they think they don't sunburn. But darker skin tones burn too. If you decide to have a beach holiday and get a deeper tan, remember to prepare your skin before you step out to the beach.

Exfoliate dead cells from your face and body; that way the tan will be more even and longer-lasting (do this twice a week).

For the first three to four days under the sun, use SPF 15 to 30 (some cosmetic companies have SPF 50 for sensitive skin) with UVA and UVB protectors. After that, when your skin has gotten used to the sun, you can lower the sunblock to SPF 15. But never go below that, even if you have a deeper skin tone.

Remember to choose a sunscreen that suits your skin type: oil-free for combination and oily skin, creamier for dry skin.

Apply a thick layer of sunscreen on your face and body and let it absorb into your skin for thirty minutes before going out under the sun.

The sun's rays are strongest between 10:00 A.M. and 4:00 P.M., so at those times you should spend your time in the shade. Don't worry, you will get tanned in the shade as well. You should wear a hat and sunglasses all the time to protect your face.

Don't lie under the sun for more than one and a half to two hours maximum a day. Drink plenty of water to keep your body temperature down.

Remember to reapply sunscreen after swimming or sweating, even if the sunblock is supposed to be water-resistant—just in case.

Use only a thin layer of sunscreen around the eye area. If a sunscreen formulation is water-resistant, the product can be brought relatively close to the eye region. However, it is vital that only a thin layer of sunscreen be applied in the eye region, extended toward the temples. A thin layer of water-resistant sunscreen will bind with the delicate under-eye skin and not travel into the eyes. Bear in mind that creams around the eyes aren't absorbed since the tissue is so thin, so a little goes a long way!

**UVA (ultraviolet A):** Long-wave solar rays. UVA rays don't necessarily cause sunburn, but they penetrate the skin more deeply and are considered the chief culprit behind wrinkling and leathering of the skin.

**UVB (ultraviolet B):** Short-wave solar rays. UVB rays are the cause of sunburn and are considered to be the main cause of basal and squamous cell carcinomas, as well as a significant cause of melanoma.

**SPF (Sun Protection Factor):** SPF measures the length of time a product protects against skin reddening from UVB, compared to how long it takes for the skin to redden without the protection. If it takes 20 minutes for the skin to redden without protection, by using SPF 15 it will take 15 times longer, or five hours. The Skin Cancer Foundation recommends using at least SPF 15, which blocks 93 percent of UVB rays. SPF 30 or higher blocks 4 percent more UVB rays than SPF 15, or 97 percent.

## AFTER SUN

After lying in the sun, always take a cool shower to freshen up and wash all the oil, dirt, sand, and sunscreen off your skin. An aloe vera— and/or chamomile-based body cleanser is good because it calms and cools the skin. Applying a thick layer of body lotion all over your body will ensure that your skin is well hydrated.

Same with the face: use a good moisturizing cream (oily skin: oil-free) to hydrate your skin. You can also use a moisturizing mask to boost moisture if you have dry skin.

For evening, you can apply a shimmery body lotion to deepen your tan and give a 3-D glow!

If you get sunburned, you should apply 0.1% cortisone cream on the area that's been burned and cover the area with a cool damp towel. A severe burn should be addressed by going to a doctor and a getting stronger medication. No more sunbathing for you!

## SELF-TANNING

Self-tanners are fast and a pretty easy way to have a sun-kissed look on your face and body. The first self-tanning lotion came onto the market in the early 1960s, but it was in the 1980s that the self-tanning market really exploded, as people's awareness of the sun's damaging effects on the skin increased.

I prefer to go a professional tanning salon, but if you want to do it yourself, here is my advice on how to make a fake tan look natural.

You must try self-tanners a couple of times and see on what areas you need the most practice: your face, neck, hands or some other area. Some products seem to create a more orange result; others are more golden yellow. I prefer tinted self-tanning lotions and gels because you can immediately see the areas where you need to blend better or add more.

There are various self-tanning formulas: cream, lotion, milky, and liquid spray, which are good for dry skin; gel-based and wipes for oilier skin; and airbrush formula for all skin types. Cream, lotion, and milky formulas take a little longer to absorb into the skin. Gel, wipes, and airbrush formulas dry faster, and liquid spray tanning is very handy, for example, to apply the product in the back. You can choose from medium (if you have fair or lighter skin) to deep color (for deeper skin tones).

1.  Before doing anything else, wax or shave any hair off your body where you want to be self-tanned (less hair equals more even result).
2.  Take a shower or bath.

3. Exfoliation is the most important step to prepare the skin for self-tanning. Use an exfoliating cream or gel to wash off dead cells and rough areas, such as on the knees, wrists, and elbows.

4. Exfoliate your face.

5. Rinse well.

6. Apply a light-formula body lotion all over your body and wait 15 to 20 minutes until it's completely absorbed into your skin.

7. Do the same on your face with face lotion.

8. Start applying the product on your legs, and move up the body in small sections. Blend. (Wear plastic gloves when applying the self-tanning product; otherwise your hands will be exposed to too much tanning product.)

9. You can ask your husband, boyfriend, or girlfriend to help with your back and also to check your whole body to see that it's even. Sometimes someone else's eyes see better.

10. After you have finished, throw the gloves away and do your face, neck, and hands (you should also do your ears if you are very fair).

11. Make sure you blend well around the eyebrows, hairline, and ears.

12. Wait 20 to 40 minutes before you dress. Don't sit down or lean on anything. I know it's hard to spend so much time doing nothing, but maybe it's time for meditation or karaoke?

13. It will take one to two hours to see the tanning result. If you think the result is too light, you can always repeat the procedures. Self-tanners stay on your skin three to seven days, depending on how many times a day you shower or bathe. But you should repeat the routine once a week.

## AIRBRUSH TANNING/TANNING SALONS

Professional tanning salons offer tanning booths and airbrush tanning.

**Jade,** *employee at the popular West Hollywood tanning salon SunStyle Tanning, www.sunstyle.la.*

When someone is coming for the first time and wants to build up a decent base tan, I recommend taking three tanning sessions in a row.
After you have the base tan, to keep up the tan, you must take one to three sessions a week, depending on how deep you want your tan to get.

Generally you do not need sunblock because the UV lamps are controlled, but if you have some very sensitive areas, I do recommend sunblock, just in case.

The best and safest way to get tanned is airbrush tanning. We offer the custom airbrush and have two different tone options to choose from. The airbrush tanning Mystic Tan is very popular. Maybe five to ten years ago the result might have been more orange than golden yellow, but today's Mystic Tan is upgraded, and we professionals know what kind of spray tanning works for any particular skin tone. For olive skin tone, more orange spray tanning looks really good, whereas on fair skin, golden brown and bronze look the best.

It takes 10 to 15 minutes maximum for Mystic Tan, one to two minutes to get airbrushed. And the spray tan lasts up to four to six days for the original Mystic Tan, and for the newer version up to 7 to 11 days.

You can also dress right after the airbrushing. You might feel a little sticky for the 20 minutes right after the application, but you won't mess up your tanning by dressing.

Before having the airbrush tanning, fully shower and exfoliate your body, don't apply any body moisturizer, and wear no deodorant. The skin must be clean before airbrushing.

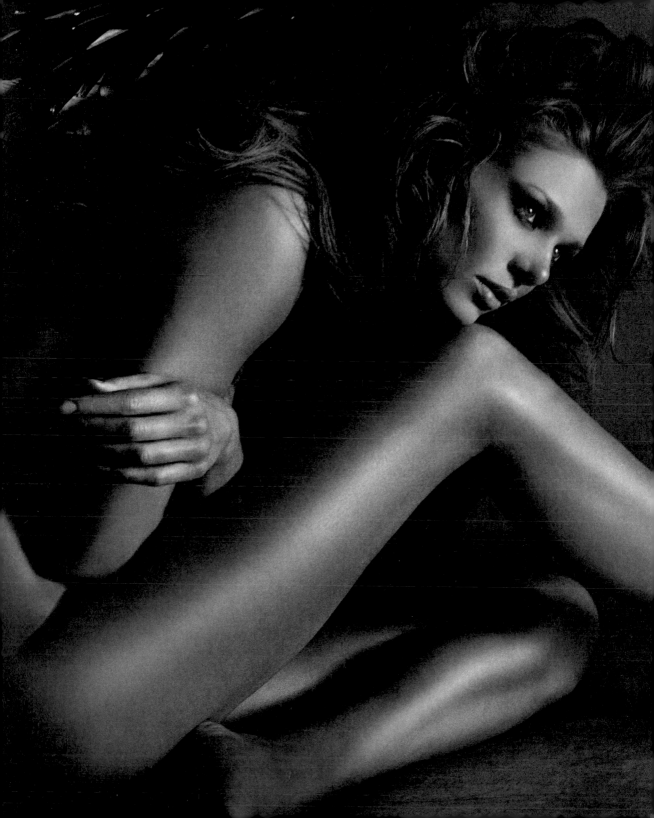

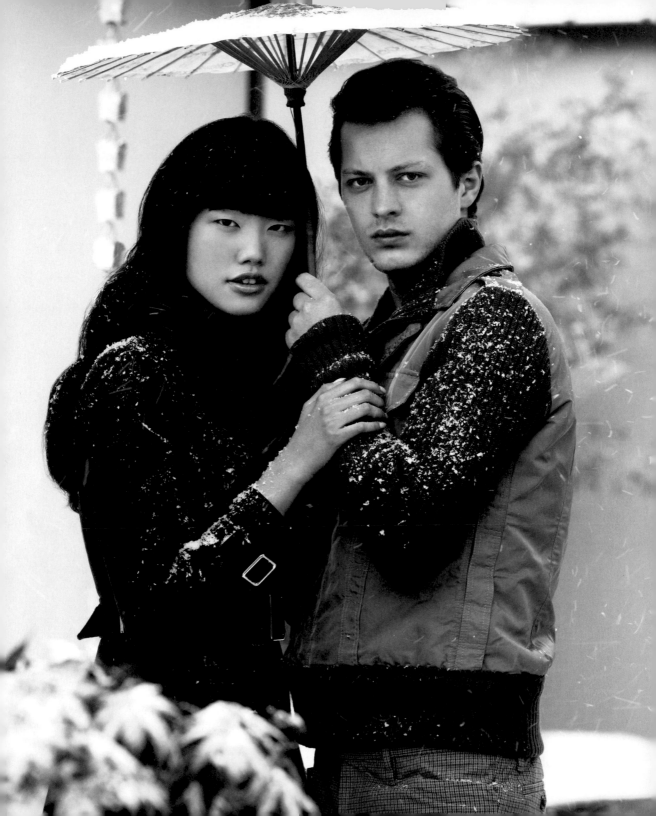

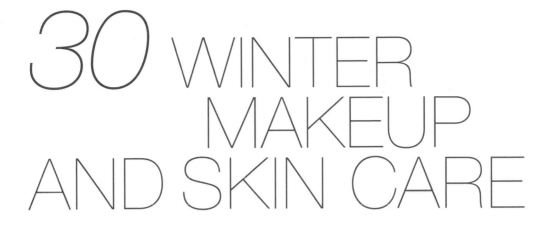

# 30 WINTER MAKEUP AND SKIN CARE

**The change of seasons is always refreshing, but winter challenges the skin and makeup more than any of the other seasons. Cold temperatures, snowy weather, heated rooms, and excessive hot showers to warm you up (which, unfortunately, also dry your skin) all make your skin need extra care and attention.**

The biggest problem is dry skin on the face, hands, and knees, and sometimes all over the body. The best advice is to moisturize. And moisturize.

Sometimes the dryness can turn into eczema. In that case you must turn to a dermatologist, who can help you choose the right skin care products. You can also use 0.1% hydracortisone once a week on the areas that are really dry, irritated, and itchy. Eczema is genetic and is most aggressive in winter.

The indoor heat along with the cold outdoor temperature makes your skin drier, no matter what your skin type is.

**Dry skin:** Use a facial serum or oil under a thicker-formula moisturizer.
**Oily Skin:** Use an oil-free serum and oil-free moisturizer.
**Combination skin:** Use oil-free products on the T-zone and a thicker moisturizer on the cheeks, which get drier in the wintertime.

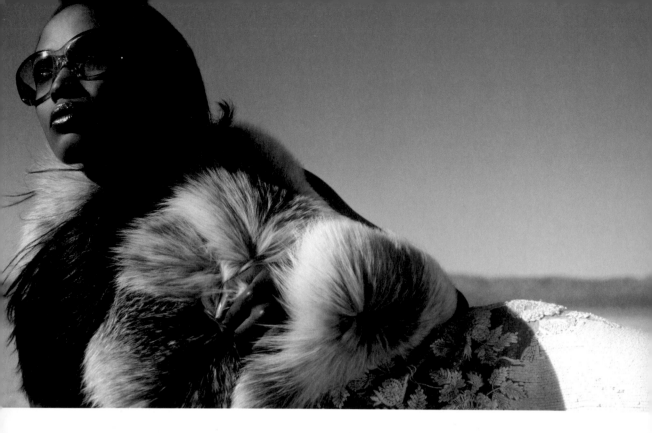

Sometimes those with oily skin should protect their skin with slightly creamier face products, especially against extremely cold temperatures and wind. Look for oil-based moisturizers (including almond, jojoba, or avocado oil) that don't clog the pores. Sometimes you might get whiteheads (tiny white cysts containing lamellated keratin that a dermatologist or esthetician can take out with a tiny needle) around your eye area or on your cheeks.

If you have dry skin, you must avoid water as much as you can; take short showers, and wash your face with a cleansing milk. And everyone should drink more water (or hot green tea) in the wintertime.

Many times dry skin gets flakes on the eyelids and cheeks and around the lip area. The best way to get rid of them is to exfoliate the skin right after showering, when the skin is still soft. After that apply a thick layer of a cream-based hydration mask all over your face. Leave it on for five minutes, then press a tissue on your face and let it absorb the mask. Don't scrub your face; just gently tap it with the tissue so you get all the extra mask off your face.

Do this in the evening, and by morning your skin will be much softer. You can use the same method on superdry lips: exfoliate your lips and the skin around them with an exfoliating cream or lip scrub (many cosmetic manufacturers make lip spa products with scrubs and various kind of balms and sealing creams).

You can also put a damp hand towel in a microwave for three minutes to heat it and then press it on your lips for a minute to soften the skin, then scrub the dead skin off gently with the towel.

Note: Scrubbing the lips with a toothbrush is really hard on them and can actually break the skin.

# MAKEUP
## BASE
Slightly richer foundations are better than tinted moisturizers because there is more to cover on your skin in the winter (uneven areas on the nose, cheeks, and eyelids).

You must use SPF/UVA/UVB protection all year round. The sun that reflects from the snow is as strong as the sun that reflects from water. So choose a day cream with at least SPF 15, or a foundation with SPF. Skin is also paler in the winter, so you must use a wintertime base.

Powder is needed all over the face for oily skin. Those with combination and dry skin should use powder on the T-area only to set the base. If your skin is dry and flaky, don't use any base product, just a face oil and your protecting SPF 15 face cream (but you can still use mascara and tinted lip balm).

## EYES
Most cosmetic companies launch autumn/winter collections full of darker shades for eye and lip makeup colors; dark grays, plums, burgundies, deep Spanish reds, and dark chocolate browns. That is because the fall/winter fashion shows give the direction to the makeup world as well. But there are no rules for which colors to use on a seasonal basis. Most of the products are matte and simply look better in winter: more dramatic and deeper hues that go hand in hand with fall/winter fashions. But remember that what works on the runway does not always work in real life.

If you love pastels in winter, go for them. Keep in mind, though, that if your

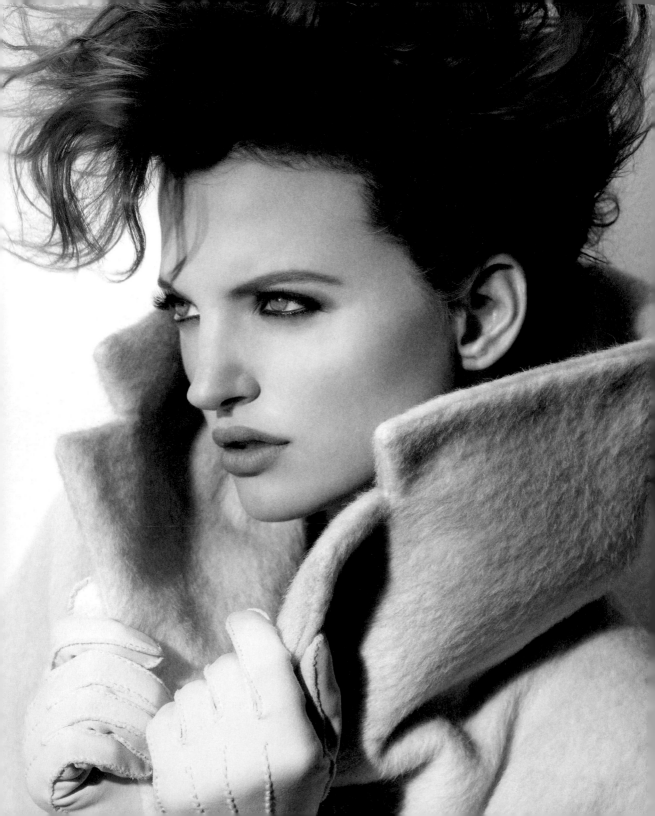

face is pale, pastel colors will create a washed-out look that is not flattering; light pastel eye and lip makeup looks better on tanned skin, which is why pastels are very popular in the summer. For a cool-tone winter look, wear deeper colors on your eyes and give your lips a matte fuchsia tone instead of light icy pink. Or use some color on your eyes and keep your lips pale (as in the photo: I gave the lashes a shocking blue wintry color!).

Mascara should be waterproof; rain, snow, and going from outdoor to indoor temperatures will make regular mascara run. You don't always have to use black mascara; try brown, blue, or green. Water-resistant eye pencil is excellent; because it's made of waxes, it will stay through the rain. Water-resistant liquid eyeliners are good but don't necessarily stay well because of their flakiness. There are some special eye makeup sealing products that you can apply on top of the eyeliner to make it hold longer. But an umbrella will do a better job in the end. I have also used water-resistant mascara as eyeliner, and sometimes it stays better than most of the real waterproof liners.

## LIPS

Cracked lips are the number one problem in winter. If your lips are superdry, skip the lipstick and use tinted lip balm, which is available in many different colors. The pigmentation is not that high, but you will get smooth, healthy-looking lips with a beautiful sheen. Make sure the balm has SPF and UVA/UVB protection. Exfoliate your lips regularly throughout the cold months. That way you will get rid of the dry flakes on the surface of your lips.

If you want a more dramatic winter look, fair skin looks really good with well-lined red lips, darker skin with well-lined deep brown or deeper cool reds. More moisturizing, richer-formula lip glosses are welcome products in the winter when the temperature drops below 0° Celsius. But on a really cold day, skip the glosses and use tinted lip balms. They protect and moisturize your lips the best.

## BLUSH

Blush is a key item to the winter makeup look. It really gives some color to your skin and wakes up your whole face. Use the powder formulas, which sit better than gel or cream blushes. The color of your blush is completely your own choice; again, if you have a cool-tone look, use pink; for a warm tone, it can be peach, warm sand, or terra-cotta. The only color I would leave out are bronzes. They really don't look great in winter.

## HANDS AND NAILS

Keep your hands moisturized. You can even sleep with cotton gloves on after applying a thick layer of hand cream to your hands. In the morning your hands and cuticles will be soft and moisturized.

Darker nail colors look trendy in the winter. You can buy a lipstick to match with your nail color because cosmetic companies launch the looks that way. It will always give a very sophisticated, mature look.

*I have oily skin in the summer, and in the winter it's dry. How can I make my skin behave in a more balanced manner from season to season?*

**Ole Henriksen answers:** It's not unusual for an oily/eruption-prone skin to become surface dry in the winter season. Two things cause this: the products used to normalize the oily skin, and the dry indoor heating plus outdoor freezing temperatures. A mistake that many people with oily skin make is to use products with too many drying agents in every product they use.

This is not necessary. It creates a dry surface mantle and potentially more oil flow below the skin surface, which can cause blemishes. Balance is the key here, using a blend of oil-free formulations with humectants such as algae, aloe vera, sorbitol, and glycerin, combined with cell-proliferating and purifying extracts such as sugar maple, sugarcane, lemon peel, and lactic acid, and finally reparative antioxidants such as vitamin C, superoxide dismutase, green tea, and African red tea. In addition, an antiblemish stick containing benzoyl peroxide, salicylic acid, bentonite, and kaolin is a must for this skin type. So the answer is to use products that contain the right blend of active ingredients and have a light texture.

*Is Vaseline good for my lips in the winter?*
Vaseline used on its own isn't thick enough to stay on the lips for long periods, but if incorporated into a lip balm formulation it works well. For people who may

not like the fact that Vaseline is a mineral oil extract, there are other extracts that work just as effectively at keeping lips soft and nourished, such as jojoba seed oil, mango seed butter, carnauba wax, and cranberry seed oil.

# TIPS

*Use a humidifier to add moisture to your indoor space if you have to use drying central heating. Put one in your bedroom, and you will notice the difference in your skin in the morning, especially when using face serum and night cream. Your skin will be softer and moister.*

*If you have very dry skin, use soap-free body wash instead of a soap bar when showering.*

*You can use a thicker-formula face cream (at least 60% oil) as your night cream. The same cream works as a deep-moisturizing face mask: just apply a thicker layer of the cream all over your face, except in the eye area. Keep it on the face for 10 to 15 minutes, and then press a tissue on the face to absorb the extra oils from the skin. Do this in the evening, and your skin will be moist, especially if you have the humidifier in your bedroom.*

*If you have sensitive skin, use a protective barrier moisturizer.*

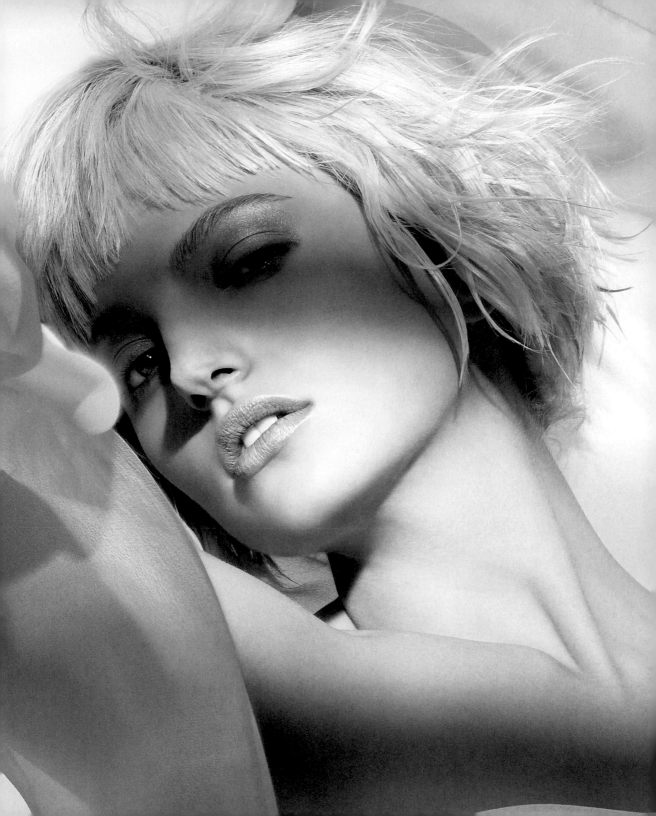

# 31 COOL-TONE MAKEUP

PHOTO: KURT ISWARIENKO/MODEL: AMANDA @ LA MODELS/HAIR: ROB TALTY

**Cool-tone makeup works with every skin color. And it always looks cool! The look in the photo is suitable for day and night. Even though the lips and eyes are both made up, the face doesn't look overloaded.**

## Get the Look

*I used a special eye base product that keeps the eye shadow from moving. I applied this to Amanda's clean eyelids before the foundation (if the moisturizer is tinted, you don't need to apply it to the eyelids).*

*I applied liquid foundation all over the face, including the lips and eyelids.*

*I applied transparent powder all over the face, including the lips and eyelids. (Use concealer if needed to cover any uneven areas on the face.)*

*I used the smaller eye shadow brush to work the light violet-blue half-shimmer shadow on the eyelids and blended it using a no. 4 brush, brushing back and forth like a windshield wiper—blending, blending!*

*I didn't use any mascara for this look, as I wanted to keep the eyes more "open" and not create the depth that mascara would have.*

*I brushed the brows and added a little brow gel to give a sheen. I didn't fill the brows, because the eye makeup would have become too "full." Another option would have been to lighten the brows two shades.*

*I tapped pink, moisturizing shimmer lipstick on Amanda's lips with a flat concealer brush.*

*I used light pink blush, very light-handed, to give brightness to her face.*

## EVENING COOL-TONE MAKEUP

This dramatic evening look will keep your look cool and mysterious.

# Get the Look

*Because evening makeup must stay on the face through dancing and partying, I used a mattifying primer on Jennifer's face before applying a light-formula oil-free liquid foundation. Remember to wait five minutes for the primer to absorb into the skin. Otherwise, the foundation might roll off.*

*I applied loose powder all over the face to keep the face matte.*

*I applied turquoise shadow to the creases of the eyes, all the way to the inner corners. I applied lighter blue shadow to the lids as well as the inside corners to lighten up the eyes.*

*I used medium-length fake eyelashes to deepen the eyes.*

PHOTO: KURT ISWARIENKO/MODEL: JENNIFER @ VISION/FUR: ROBERTO CAVALLI

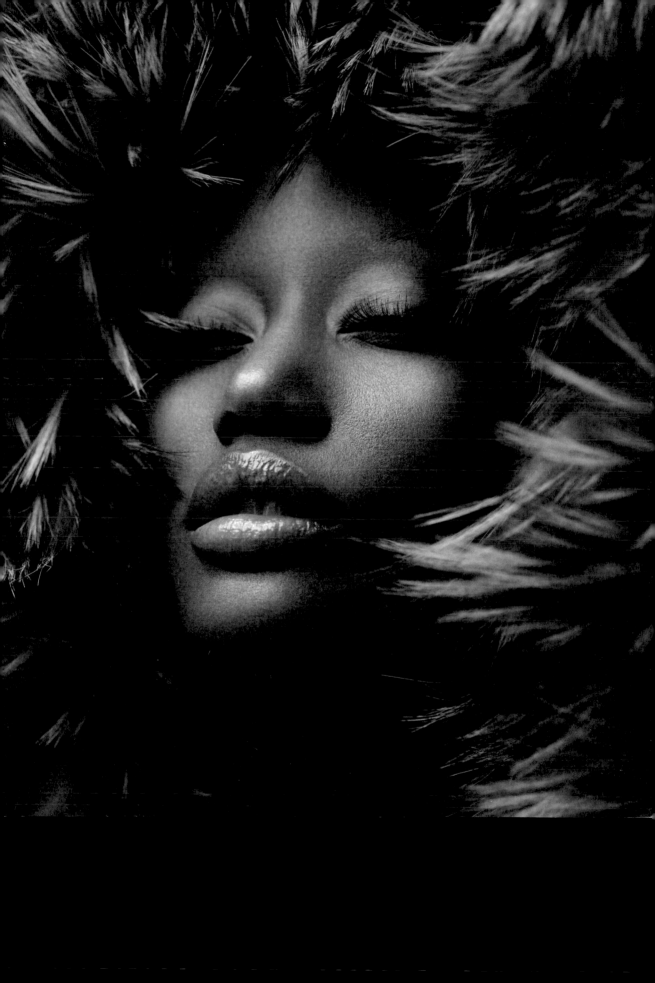

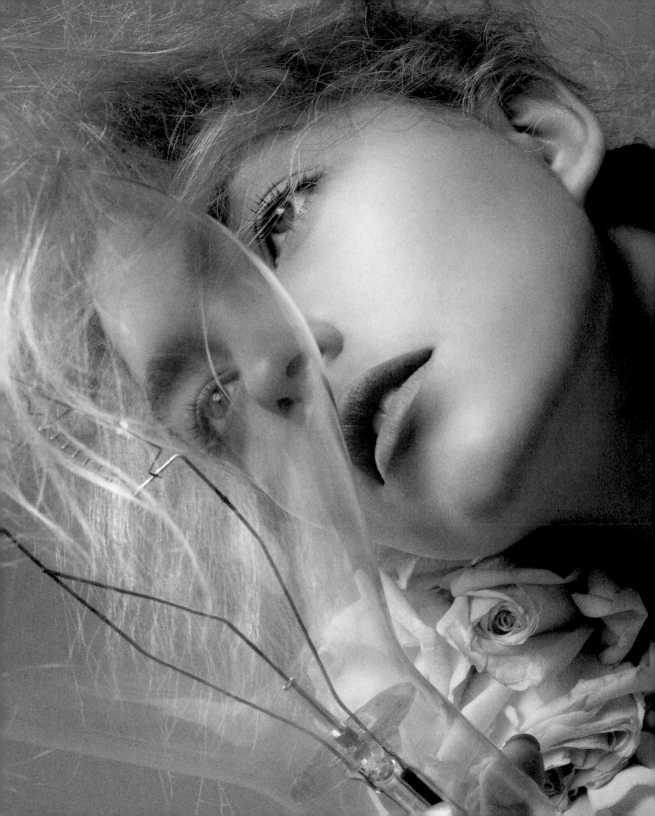

*I then applied clear cream lip gloss.*

*I kept the brows natural; otherwise the makeup would have gone overboard.*

## ONE-SPOT COOL-TONE MAKEUP

Bright fuchsia lips are very dominant, and you don't want almost any other makeup, because the bright color really gives the face the color and attitude you are looking for. A great color for the spring!

# Get the Look

*I applied just a little moisturizer to Arizona's face, and lip balm to her lips.*

*I applied tinted moisturizer and loose powder to her face and lips.*

*I used a fuchsia lip liner to create this look. I lined the lips and filled them with the liner.*

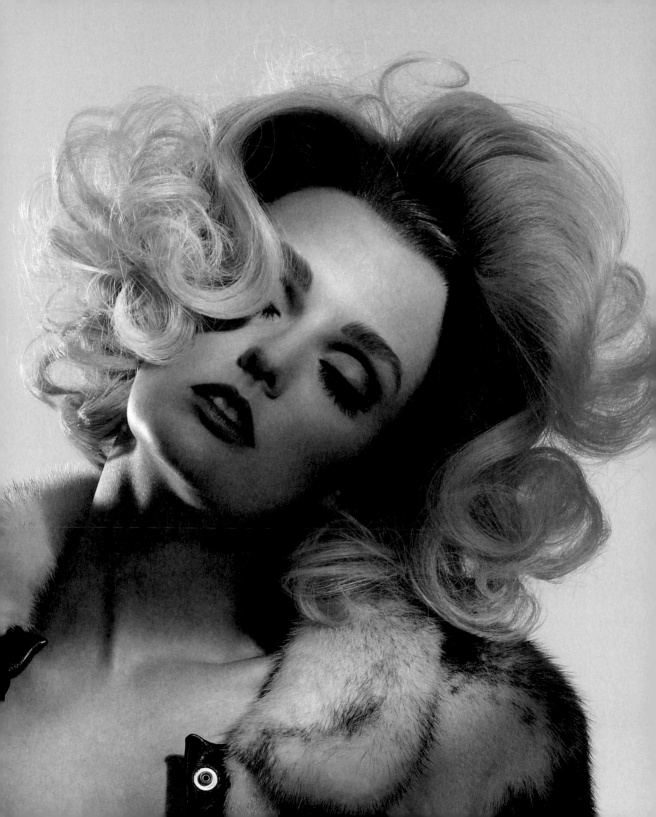

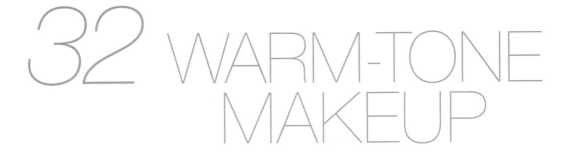

# 32 WARM-TONE MAKEUP

This color group creates a warm feel on your face. All the colors contain red, which keeps them on the warm side of the color chart. Warm brown, peach, coral, orange, warm-tone red, and red brick/terra-cotta are very popular and some of the most-sold colors in eye shadows, blushes, lipsticks, and glosses. They're easy to mix and match!

## Get the Look

**Tools:** *oil-free liquid foundation, concealer, and transparent loose powder*

*I wanted to create the early-'70s look on Lydia's face with all warm-tone colors.*

*I used a medium dark brown matte eye shadow on the crease and the lash line and blended well. A liquid liner on the lash line deepened the look.*

*I then applied fake eyelashes.*

*I used a light peach-based nude color on the lips and warm peach blush on the apples to give the face warmth.*

*Then I brushed the brows.*

PHOTO: KURT ISWARIENKO/MODEL: LYDIA HEARST/HAIR: ROB TALTY/STYLE: LEILA BABOI

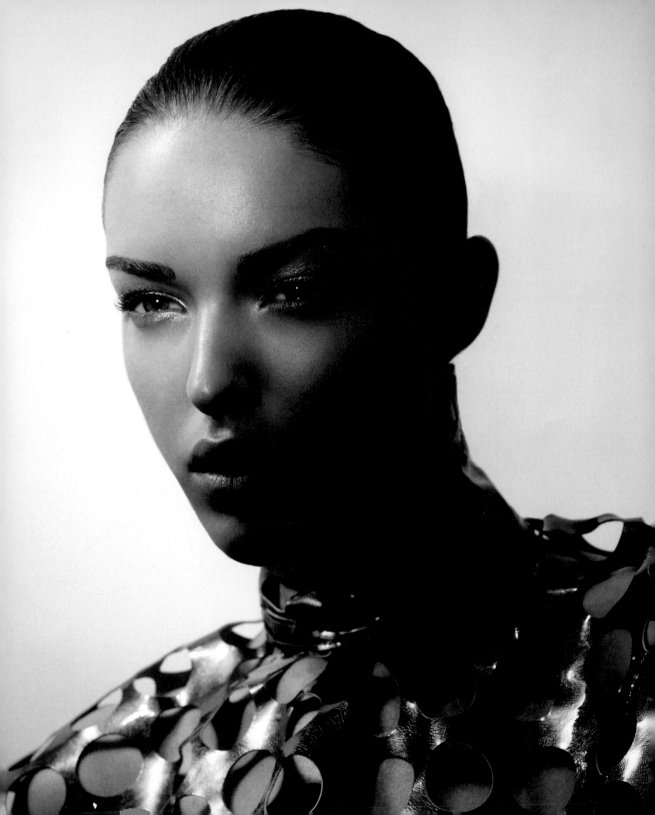

# 33 METALLIC MAKEUP

**Metallic makeup always looks cool. Metallics really work better for evening. Apply to the lips or eyes.**

## GOLD

Gold eye shadow looks beautiful without any other eye makeup. Make sure the shadow has a rich pigmentation. Also apply the shadow inside the corners of your eyes; it opens up the eyes by reflecting the light. Gold liner also looks amazing on any skin tone from fair to dark.

CELEBRITY NAIL STYLIST
JENNA HIPP CREATED
THESE FABULOUS GOLDEN
METALLIC NAILS USING
MINX NAIL SYSTEM
(MINXNAILS.COM), WHERE
A PIECE OF A SOLID FILM
WITH AN ADHESIVE BACK
WAS PLACED ON EVERY
FINGERNAIL AND THEN
HEATED WITH THE HELP
OF A HEATLAMP.

## Bronze

Strong, bronzy lips are stunning when you are tanned or have medium or dark skin. You can use a bronze lip liner; line and fill the lips with the liner as I did, but keep the eye makeup on the more natural side. To get a more natural result on fair skin, tap sheer bronze lipstick on your lips with your finger. Bronze also lip glosses look more natural.

PHOTO: KURT ISWARIENKO/MODEL: SARAH @ LA MODELS/HAIR: LOUISE MOON

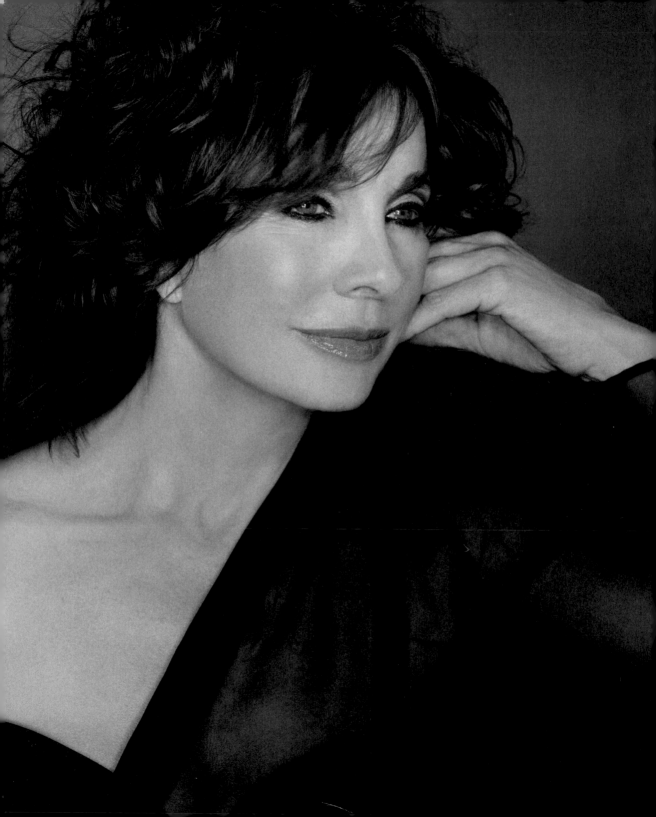

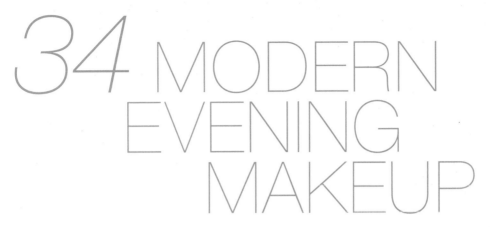

# 34 MODERN EVENING MAKEUP

**When I met the talented and beautiful actress Anne Archer for the first time to do her makeup, I was so excited, because I had always loved her movies. Anne's skin is in excellent condition, and it made my work quite easy.**

I wanted to create something very classy but at the same time an ultramodern makeup look that would enhance Anne's beautiful eyes. This evening look also works perfectly if you have an important dinner engagement because the focus is on the eyes. When you drink, you can wear red lipstick, but for dinner, it's a different story, because you drink, eat, and talk and your lip makeup will fade, whether you want it to or not. So keep the volume in the eyes and the lips more natural but still defined and gorgeous!

## Get the Look

*I prepped Anne's skin with a moisturizer and primer.*

*I applied compact foundation very lightly all over the face, remembering the lips and eyelids. I blended well from the jawline down to avoid any visible lines between the neck and face.*

*I powdered the eyelids. They must be totally matte and dry for this look.*

*I started with matte gray eye shadow. (Gray works very well with black kohl, giving the eyes a 3-D effect.) I used a small eye shadow brush to apply the gray to the lash lines and blend it well up to the crease (not higher).*

*I applied black kohl on the upper lash line and blended it a little by using a small round-shape eye brush, avoiding a too-harsh line.*

*I also used the kohl as an inside liner on the lower lids. It gives that instant evening look for the eyes.*

*I curled Anne's lashes before I applied two layers of black thickening mascara.*

*I lined the lips, keeping them natural and in a cool tone. I lined and filled the lips with the liner, and on top of that I applied a sheer cool-tone lipstick that had a beautiful shine. This also kept the lips from looking too dry.*

*I used a light icy pink shimmer blush for a little highlighting on her cheeks. Remember, a little bit goes a long way.*

## TO TAKE ALONG IN THE EVENING

**Compact cream-powder** for touch-ups (comes with a mirror)
**Lip liner and lipstick**
**Black kohl,** because it will fade, so make sure to check your inside liner at some point in the evening
**A couple of Q-tips.** You should always carry them as your SOS tools; with them you can clean and fix the corners of your eyes and lips as well as your eyelids

# Anne Archer, Actress

*I have dry skin, so my daily routine for skin care and makeup begins with cleansing with a gentle milk cleanser, and I don't use any water. Then I wipe off with Kleenex and follow with a toner. I also clean often with good old Cetaphil. It's so gentle, and also cheap. At night I use a product distributed by DermoGenesis and made by Environ called C-Quence, a fluid that gradually gets rid of spotting and lines. It's an amazing product that one uses every night forever! It's made in South Africa by a renowned dermatologist, and I was introduced to it through an esthetician in London when I was performing in* The Graduate *in the West End. I use a heavy night cream on top of that. In the morning I cleanse again, and for my moisturizer I use two Epicuran products that I mix together, Colostrum Cream Serum and Discovery (a rejuvenation therapy product).*

*My favorite foundation is Chanel's Vitalumière. I like Laura Mercier's powders. I do various shadows on my eyes, in a very light way: a powder line, mascara, and lipstick. For eye shadows I use a lot of Chantcaille products. For the night I make my eyes smokier, and if I have to be more glam I add some individual fake lashes.*

*When I'm filming, I bring some specific makeup products to my makeup artist to use. I bring Chanel's foundation, Smashbox's Brow Tech Powder, and Lancôme's Bronzelle lip liners. It's important that the makeup and especially the lip liner look very natural, because everything on camera is exaggerated. I also bring Laura Mercier's translucent powder and eye-brightening powder.*

*Special makeup tricks I have noticed over the years that really work: I extend my eye shadow very subtly partially over the brow bone and out to the side to give the illusion that my eyes are almond shaped—better for me.*

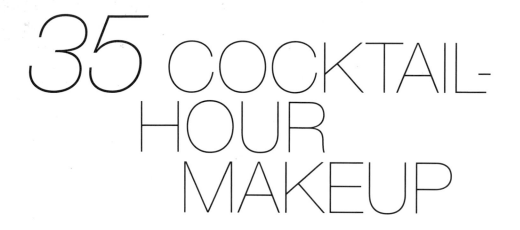

# 35 COCKTAIL-HOUR MAKEUP

**Cocktail-hour makeup is all about matte skin and red matte lips, which together create a perfect early-evening look. The look is sophisticated and has a hint of old-time glamour.**

You may have read that you can't wear red lipstick to cocktail parties because it won't stay on your lips. Well, it doesn't if you apply the lipstick on your bare lips without applying any base first. There are other little tricks that will make sure you will still be wearing the same lipstick when it's time to leave the party. Because red lips are very dominating, the eye makeup is only a black liquid eyeliner and black mascara.

## Get the Look

*I applied concealer with a concealer brush to cover any uneven areas of the skin (under the eyes, around the nose, cheeks).*

*I applied liquid foundation all over the face, using a sponge. I also applied foundation on the eyelids and lips to provide a great base for eye and lip makeup.*

PHOTO: DANIELA FEDERICI/MODEL: NOELLE ROQUE @ ELITE/HAIR: DAMIEN MONZILLO/PUBLISHED IN LA CONFIDENTAL MAGAZINE

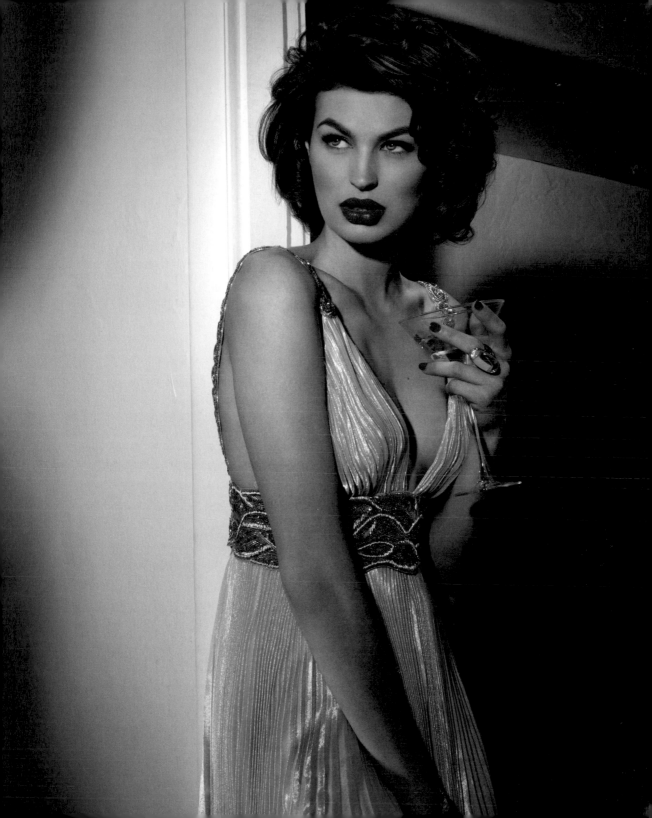

*I applied loose powder all over the face, including the lips and eyelids.*

*I started the makeup on the lips, lining and filling the lips with lip liner. If your lips feel dry after powdering, you can apply a very small amount of Vaseline to your lips before laying on the color. Make sure that your lips are symmetric after you finish. Red lips don't look good if the sides of the lips are not even. It's easy to correct this with the lip liner. Make sure your lip liner is not a cool tone if your lipstick is a warm-tone red. Don't overpaint your lips with the lipstick; it's more about tapping the color on the top of the lined and filled lips than painting them. Otherwise the lipstick won't stay and will run off after your first drink. Lip stains are also a good option for a long-lasting lip makeup, but their problem is that they look very dry.*

*I applied black liquid eyeliner to the roots of the lashes. My favorite is the pencil eyeliner kind because it's easier to control and the brush is always wet with color. Plus, you can carry the product in your handbag (just in case something happens).*

*I applied natural-size fake eyelashes; first I applied one coat of black mascara, then I set the lashes and glued them into place. If you can see the little strips of fake lashes, tap black liner on top of the strip.*

*I used eyebrow pencil to fill the brows. I am a huge fan of pencils because you will get a more natural eyebrow look than with a matte eye shadow or brow gel.*

*I used a matte bronzer to contour the model's face with a big blush brush.*

### Why do you use a liquid foundation instead of a tinted moisturizer for this look?

Liquid foundation creates a better base for a matte skin look, as well as for the eye and lip makeup.

### Why do you fill the lips with lip liner?

Lip makeup stays much better that way. It's like building a wall around the lips. But you must remember not to add too much lipstick; otherwise it will run over like a big wave.

### I have oily skin. How can I create a truly matte evening look?

Do a minifacial at home before applying oil-free liquid foundation: exfoliate your skin, use a clay mask that sucks the oil off your skin, and use a primer that is oil-free and designed to keep the face matte. Then start your makeup. Remember to take the blotting papers and pressed powder with you—just in case.

### My lips are dry. How can I make this cocktail makeup work for me?

Exfoliate your lips (see more about the lip spa on page 195) and use a lot of lip balm the night before the event.

---

*TIP* Lip stains are also excellent for a longlasting lip makeup when you eat and drink.

---

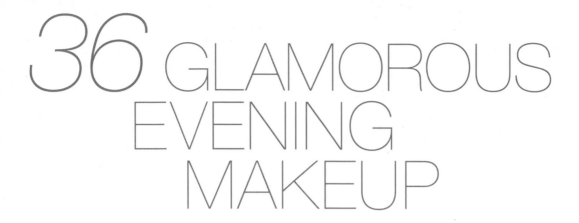

# 36 GLAMOROUS EVENING MAKEUP

I have worked with many actors for their gala events in Hollywood, and I know how to make their makeup last from the red carpet to the parties afterward. I created two different looks, just by changing the lipstick color. Other than that, the rest of the makeup is the same. What a difference a simple lipstick color makes! This '50s-inspired evening look is for those of you who want to look classy and elegant. The makeup is full, but it stays together without looking too made up when you keep the eyes without any dramatic shadow, the skin matte, and the face without theatrical contouring.

## PREPARATION

1. Exfoliate the skin and lips.
2. Use a mask appropriate for your skin type.
3. Moisturize.
4. Use a primer-filler to take care of any fine lines and visible pores.

PHOTOS 221, 223: COLIN ANGUS/MODEL: DIANA GEORGIE @ CLICK/HAIR: ROB TALTY/NAILS: BETH FRICKE/STYLING: HEIDI MEEK/FUR: SOMBER FURS

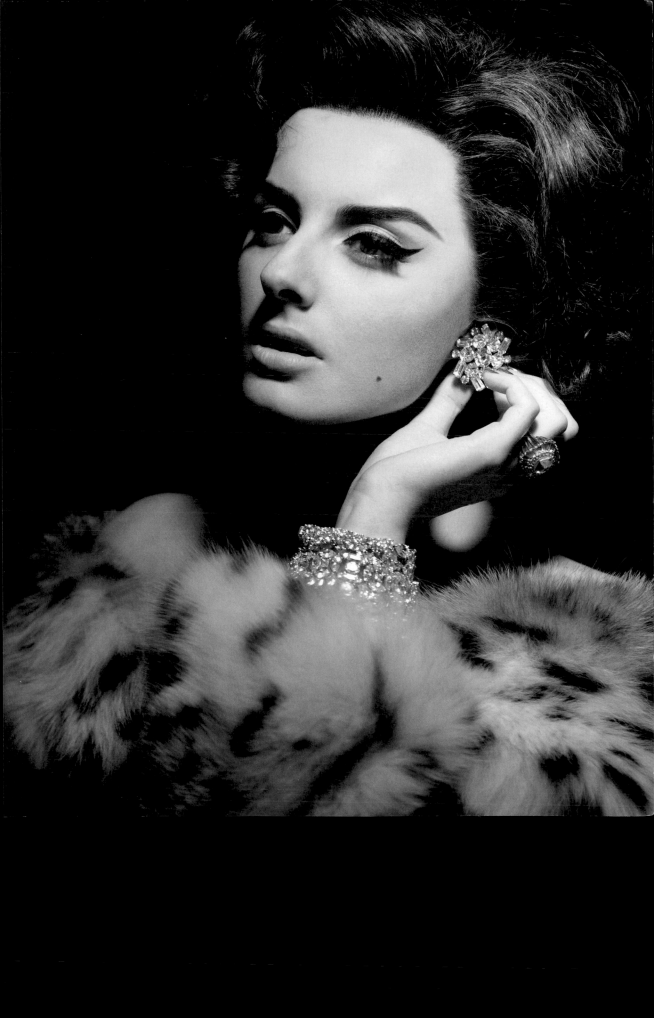

# Get the Look

*I used concealer where needed.*

*I applied liquid foundation and then loose powder all over the face, neck, and décolleté.*

*I applied ivory matte eye shadow all over the lids to lighten up the eyes and light brown matte shadow in the crease.*

*I used an automatic pencil formula of black liquid eyeliner. (It's the easiest for you as well.) I made the liner thicker from the middle of the eye to the outer corner and created wings to lift the eyes. Here's the trick: powder the liner after it has dried completely and redo the liner. Just as with the long-lasting lip makeup trick in the cocktail-hour makeup chapter, this makes the liner last longer.*

*I then applied black mascara and medium-size, natural-length thickened fake eyelashes.*

*I made the eyebrows stronger, and Diana's natural arch helped me create that '60s-inspired brow look. I used brown matte eye shadow and the brow brush.*

*On the lips: I used a natural-color creamy matte lipstick. I line the lips carefully and filled the lips with the pencil. I applied the lipstick and then pressed a tissue on the lips, powdered them, and applied another coat of lipstick.*

*I used a slightly darker blush (sand color) just under Diana's cheeks to contour her face.*

*And now you are ready for the cameras and partying!*

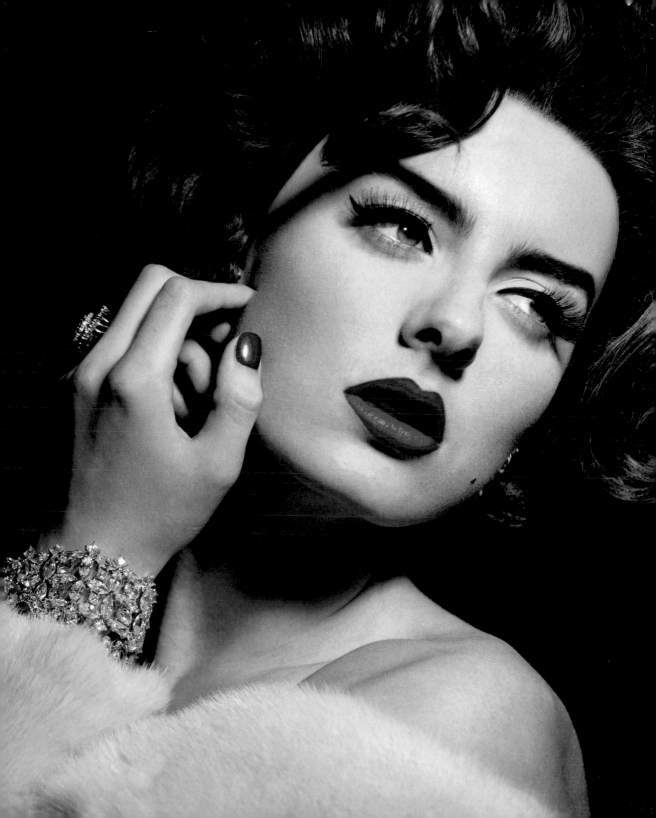

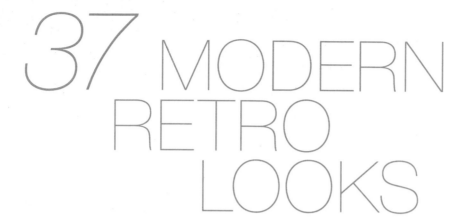

# 37 MODERN RETRO LOOKS

I love bringing retro makeup alive in a modern way. As an artist, I often get my inspiration from the past. If a fashion editor shows me a dress with a late-'30s vibe, it gives me a flash of what I can do with the makeup. Certain colors or fabrics can also give a strong retro vision. It's so inspiring and rewarding.

This look is inspired by the late-'20s silent actress Louise Brooks and the '80s pop singer Corinne Drewery of Swing Out Sister, all with a modern twist. Kind of '20s meets the '80s.

## Get the Look

*I used tinted moisturizer and transparent loose powder to create a good, natural-looking base.*

*I thickened and shaped the brows with a black matte eye shadow and an eyebrow brush to give the '80s dramatic brow.*

*Then I applied black mascara and a little Vaseline on the lids to catch the light.*

PHOTO: KURT ISWARIENKO / MODEL: KAROLINA NEVIA @ PHOTOGENICS/ STYLING: RIKU/NAILS: BETH FRICKE

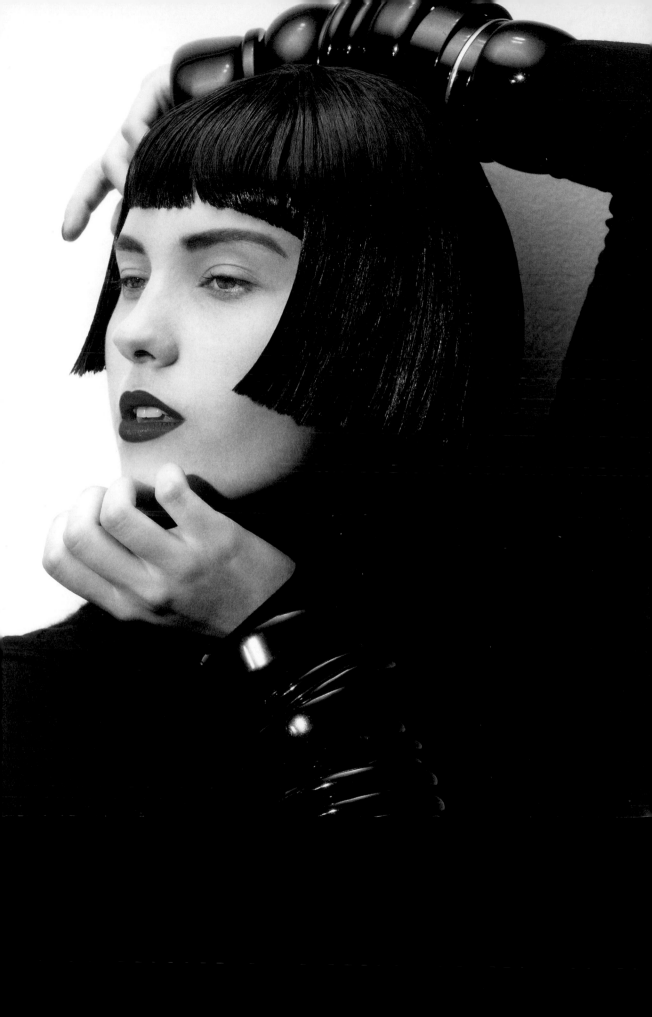

I lined the lips and filled them with a true red. (I didn't want the lips to have a small Cupid shape, so I followed the model's natural lip line.)

# Get the Look

A Hollywood icon, the actress Rebecca De Mornay is one of the true classic beauties. Rebecca is a modern, fashionable woman, and I wanted to give her a hint of '60s European bohemian style with a strong liquid eyeliner and pale lips, sort of a modern Bardot.

I applied a moisturizing cream and an eye-area gel.

Then I applied a light-reflecting primer, a liquid, oil-free foundation, concealer, and transparent loose powder.

I applied liquid liner with an easy-to-use automatic liner pencil. (It travels well and gives a good, steady result.)

I made the liquid liner extend on the outer corners as "wings" to create that '60s look.

I then applied black mascara and natural-length fake lashes.

I left the lips matte and nude.

Keep the eyebrows very natural, because otherwise the makeup will look too busy.

PHOTO: RANDEE ST. NICHOLAS/MODEL: REBECCA DE MORNAY/HAIR: BERTRAND W.

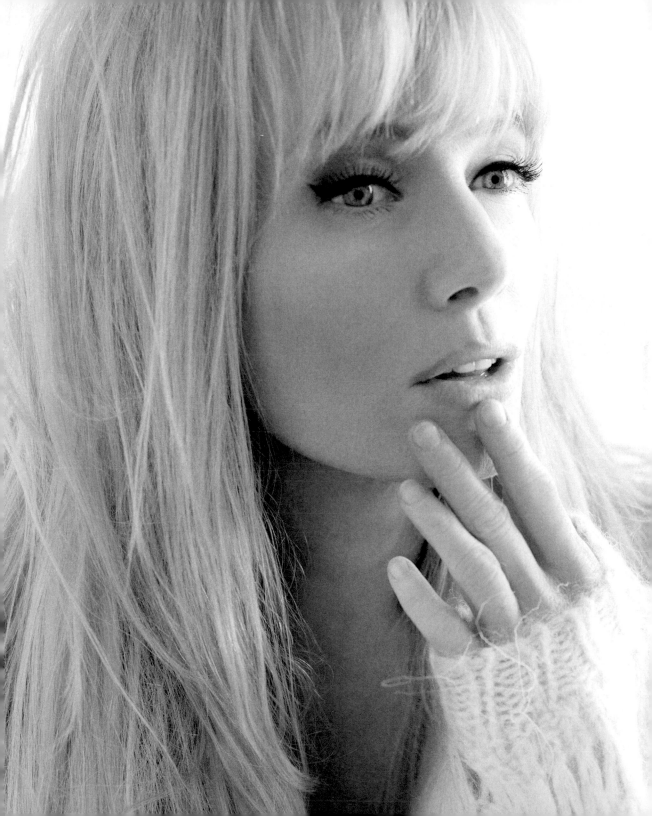

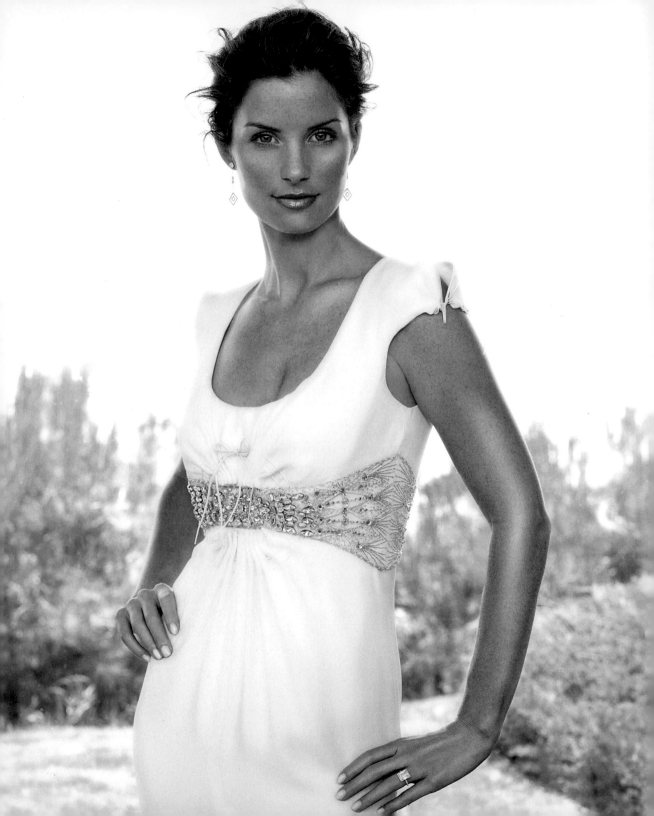

# 38 BRIDAL MAKEUP

PHOTO: PASCAL DEMEESTER/MODEL: KARA @ WILHELMINA/HAIR: KEIKO HAMAGUCHI/PUBLISHED IN LA WEDDINGS

**Your wedding day is one of the biggest, happiest, and most memorable days of your life!**

You're planning your wedding: location, guest list, catering, decorations, flowers, and yes, of course, the dress that is the biggest-kept secret until the actual wedding day—but then you need to decide which direction you want to go with your hair and makeup. The dress, the location (indoors or outdoors), and the style or theme of the wedding will give an idea and direction for your hairdo and makeup. It's a good idea to hire a makeup artist, hair stylist, and manicurist, a professional beauty team to bring out the best of you on that very special day. I created three different bridal makeups that are very different but all elegantly beautiful.

## MODERN CLASSY BRIDE

**Location:** *Outside a chapel on the beach in Florida*
**Time:** *6:00 P.M., close to sunset*

The gown is classic white and simply beautiful. Because the wedding is outdoors, we decided to go with a natural, minimalist look that would make the bride's skin glow. The makeup is based on the bride's beautifully tanned caramel-colored skin. First I applied a thicker-formula body cream to moisturize and hydrate the skin. (The bride exfoliated her body in the shower beforehand to wash away all dead cells and create a more beautiful skin surface, glowing and healthy-looking.)

To get a deeper tan, you can take a couple of tanning-bed treatments and a spray tanning a couple of days before the wedding. Or maybe your wedding will be in a sunny location and you can tan yourself at the beach for one to three days. But be careful with the sun; use 30 SPF with UVA and UVB. The hair design is a modern updo, good for an outside wedding because of the possible wind and humidity. Before I started doing the bride's face, the hair stylist blow-dried the hair and set it on big rollers.

I applied a cream-based hydration mask on the bride's face for 15 minutes to moisturize and relax her skin (the skin gets dry, especially after taking sun) and at the same time did a hand massage to relax the excited, nervous bride. (If the bride has oily skin, a clay-based mask should be used; for combination skin the clay mask should be used only on the skin that is oily, usually the T-zone.)

I wiped the mask off the face using wet cloths and toner, with the help of cotton swabs. I repeated the toner step to make sure the skin was clean of the mask.

I exfoliated the lips and applied a thick layer of lip balm.

I followed with the skin care products: eye-area gel, light facial serum, and daytime moisturizer with SPF with 15 UVA and UVB. I waited 10 minutes for all the skin care products to absorb into the skin.

I plucked any obvious hairs from above or below the brow line.

I covered any uneven areas on the face with a concealer. I chose a light-formula gel-based tinted moisturizer that really made it look as though the bride was not wearing any makeup on her face. I loved the dewy look on her because her skin was drier. I powdered only the eyelids.

Because the wedding ceremony can be very emotional, it's important to apply makeup to endure through the tears of laughter and movements. Some brides are more emotional than others, so remember to ask the bride if she easily gets tears in the corners of her eyes.

I kept the eyes very neutral. Because of the humidity, I used a cream eye shadow in light bronze that would reflect the light of the sunset, just enough to give the eyes a glam feel.

I applied the shadow by tapping it all over the lid with my ring finger, up to the crease, and blended it well. Cream shadow is also good if the bride shows some tears, because the cream formula contains silicon, which repels water.

I applied one coat of a special lash primer that separates the lashes as well as making them water-resistant. I applied two coats of black mascara and curled the lashes with a heating curler.

I didn't use any fake eyelashes because the look was very pure, natural, and modern. I filled the brows with a brow pencil, very light-handed, brushed the brows, and set them with a brow gel.

I applied a cream blush in warm peach that reflected the light beautifully. You can tap the blush on with a sponge, foundation brush, or just your fingers.

I use a special lip primer and then tapped a little foundation on the lips to make the skin color even.

I lined the lips, tapped the lipstick on with a lip brush, and finished the application with a light caramel-colored gloss.

After the bride changed into her wedding gown, I applied a light touch of a creamy body lotion to give more sheen on the skin. I didn't use a body bronzer, which doesn't work well with her white gowns.

The mani-pedicure was very natural, with sheer nail polish. Remember to give your bridesmaids a lip gloss, blotting papers, Q-tips, tissue, and a compact powder container with a mirror to hold for your touch-ups.

## MODERN GLAMOROUS

**Location:** *A beautiful hotel ballroom*

**Time:** *Noon*

This wedding gown is made of feathers and is a nontraditional color, but it is absolutely stunning. When the bride walks with the gown on, the feathers move with the air in a breathtaking way. The look for the face and hair was modern glamour.

I used a light-textured body cream all over.

I applied a clay mask for 15 minutes to absorb the oil from the skin (don't ever apply a mask around the eyes, because it's too heavy for the sensitive eye area if you don't have oily skin).

The bride washed the mask off with cool water (cool water keeps the pores closed). I sprayed a grease-relief toner on two cotton swabs and tapped them all over the skin to close the pores and hydrate the skin. Then I applied an eye-area gel and a light-formula oil-free moisturizer. I waited five minutes before I applied an

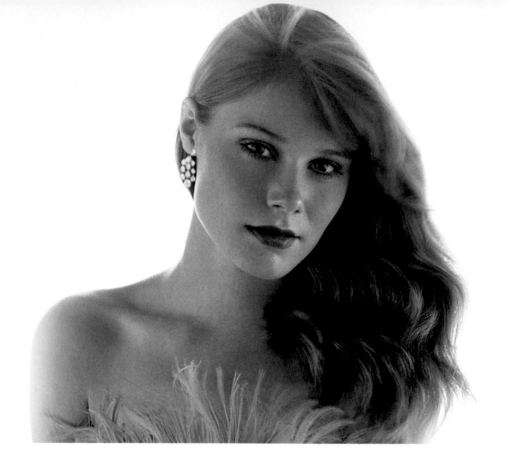

antishine primer to build up a barrier between the skin and foundation and keep the skin matte for a longer time.

I plucked the eyebrows to correct their shape.

The bride is very fair, so I used a yellow-based ivory oil-free liquid foundation. I then applied a yellow-based ivory-tone concealer to cover uneven areas on the face, blending well. I used a transparent matte loose powder over the foundation powder all over the face to set the base and keep the skin matte.

All makeup is matte. I applied an ivory-color eye shadow all over the lid to open the eyes. (Don't apply white under the brow bone, because it will look too made up, and often it will make your eyes look even smaller. The crease is the border.) The bride had naturally curved lashes, so I just applied two coats of water-resistant brown-black mascara. Between the applications I brushed the lashes with a lash brush to get rid of any clumps (you can also use a metallic lash comb).

I filled the brows with a matte light brown eye shadow and brushed the brows.

Lip primer is a great product to use for events like this, because you really want your lip makeup to stay and to not have to worry if the lipstick is going to stay or not. I applied foundation on top of the primer and powdered the lips lightly to create a perfect surface for long-lasting lip makeup. I tapped on a cooler-tone dark berry–colored lipstick with a lip brush, pressed a tissue on the lips, and applied a second layer to ensure that the color would stay on the lips during the wedding.

I used just a hint of blush in a very natural pink tone to give the face warmth.

The hair is old Hollywood glam: '40s-style waves, but with a modern twist. Yiotis curl-ironed the hair and brushed it out to get the wavy design. He used a little bit of special hair-smoothing cream to tame small flying hairs and then finished the do with a light-textured hair spray.

## RETRO

**Location:** *A 1950s-style villa*
**Time:** *4:00 P.M.*

The bride loves 1950s styles and wants to create the whole wedding around that theme. Her wedding gown is a vintage piece.

The bride has normal-combination skin, which means that the T-zone is oily and the rest of the face is dry. I applied a tightening, lifting face mask for 15 minutes to give the skin an extra boost. I also applied eye treatment pads (you leave them on for 15 minutes and peel them off; they're also great when you're traveling, or anytime you need a quick boost under the eyes). After the pad treatments, I applied a lift serum that tightened up the pores and gave the skin an instant lift. On top of that I applied a light-textured day cream. The skin looks relaxed and glowing.

Nina's brows were naturally a perfect '50s shape, so I really didn't have to pluck them.

I used a yellow-based concealer under the eyes, just on the inside corners, on the darkest areas. Then I applied a lifting foundation that is very light, but in a cream formula that gives a little bit more coverage. A lip primer is a must. I used a transparent loose powder all over the face to create a matte effect, but was very light-handed, especially under the eyes.

I created the cat's-eye look with black liquid liner, fake lashes, ivory and medium matte brown shadows, and strong retro-feeling brows.

The bride's damp hair was set in traditional velvet rollers and each section was sprayed with a special setting lotion. After 45 minutes under a dryer, the hair was brushed out, teased, and set in the glam '50s-style waves and curls. Taru finished the hair with hairspray and shine spray.

## OLE HENRIKSEN ON WEDDING PREP

*My wedding day is approaching, and I have a red pimple in the middle of my forehead. Is there anything I can do?*

We have been faced with this problem many times at my spa, getting a bride ready the day before her wedding. The best way to release inflammation is with a warm compress applied directly to the pimple. Gently press with either a warm flat sponge or a piece of soft cotton and hold firmly in place, don't rub or glide it on the blemish. Repeat at least two to three times. Now wrap supersoft tissue around each index finger and begin to gently press around the outer perimeters of the pimple. Press upward while gently removing the pus. Press and then let go, then press again until you see a little blood, which indicates that all the infection has been removed. When you are done, drench a small piece of cotton with alcohol and press the cotton toward the pimple. This will ensure that the pimple will not reinfect. Apply the same solution an hour later. No makeup, concealer, or cream should be applied on the spot for at least eight hours if possible. Exfoliants should be avoided for several days afterward. After eight hours, makeup can be applied.

*How many times should I see an esthetician before my wedding to look my best?*

Start six weeks prior to the wedding with a deep-cleansing treatment; follow two weeks later with a microdermabrasion treatment; and then two or three days before the wedding have a hydrating/firming treatment void of any extractions, unless there is an emergency blemish to be dealt with.

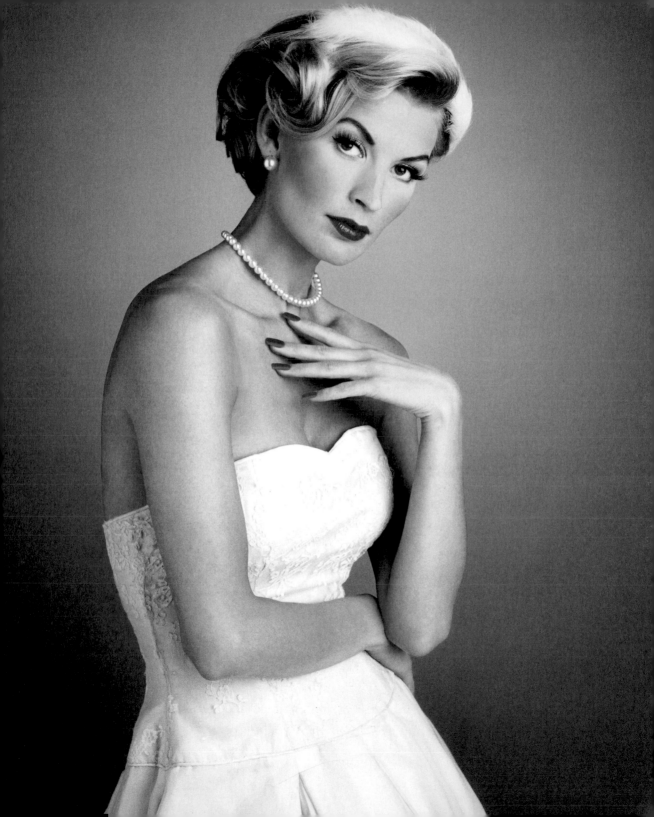

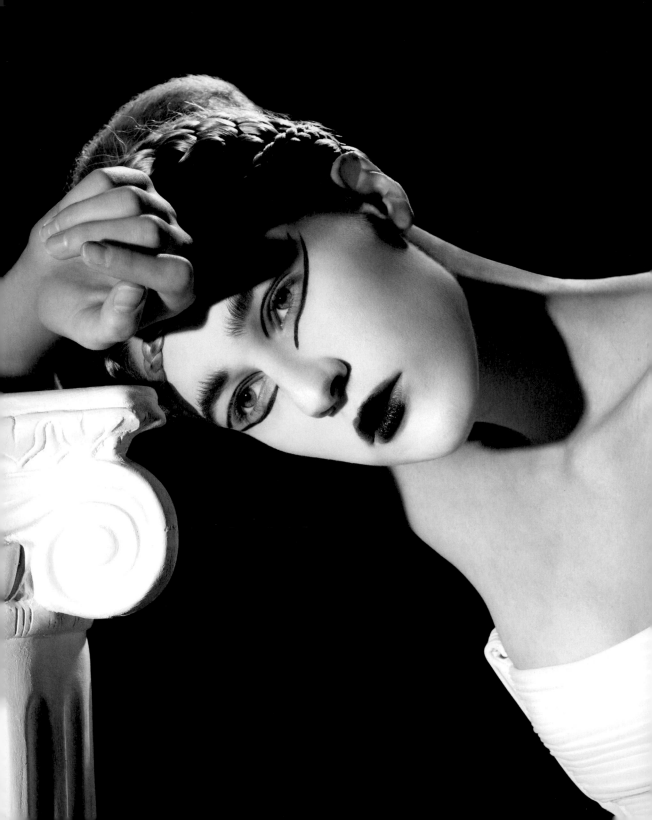

PHOTO: GITTE MELDGAARD/MODEL: AUTUMN @ PHOTOGENICS/HAIR: YIOTIS/NAILS: JENNA HIPP/STYLING: HEIDI MEEK

# 39
# INTERNATIONAL LOOKS

**Makeup has played a big part in human history. Every corner of the world and all people have their own perceptions of beauty, which are based on their own cultural history.**

## ATHENS LOOK

Greek beauty is based on the mythology of Aphrodite, the goddess of love and beauty. Homerian Greeks are believed to have used little makeup, but later Greek women used paints and washes (usually rose and white) to color the skin. The white color was usually white lead, which for more than two thousand years would whiten women's faces, destroy their complexions, and even result in premature death. The rouge was often made of vegetable substances such as mulberry. Rouged cheeks were normally accompanied by rouged lips, though many times the lips alone were colored, sometimes quite heavily. Dark, painted eyebrows were a very important beauty concept in Greek culture. Some women even wore false eyebrows. Egyptian kohl and sometimes ordinary soot or lampblack was used in eye makeup. Both women and men adored blond hair, and it was fashionable to lighten the hair by washing it with a special bleaching ointment and sitting under the sun for hours to get the golden result. Fragrant oils were used in the hair.

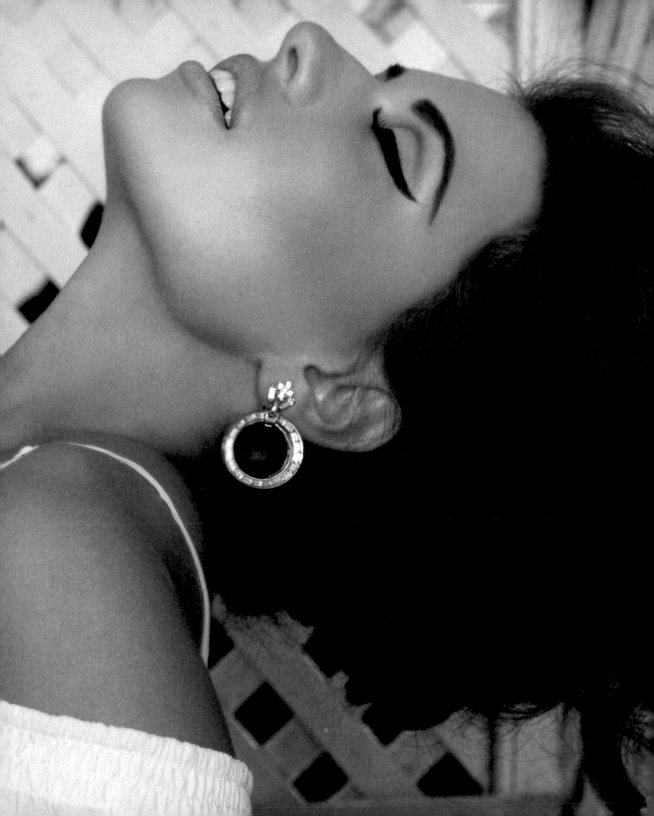

Olive, sesame, almond, and palm oils as well goose fat and butter were used in cosmetics.

The makeup I did for this picture is a mix of a traditional Greek beauty concept and Greek stage makeup.

## NAPLES LOOK

The Italians had Venus, their own version of Aphrodite. But it's very much the Italian film divas who have defined our perception of this nation's female beauty: Sophia Loren, Gina Lollobrigida, Anna Magnani, and Claudia Cardinale. Their heavily lined cat's eyes captivated audiences around the world, and the Italian look was born. It's very much based on the '60s-style thick black liquid eyeliner, fake lashes, dark Mediterranean brows, and matte foundation lips, not to mention the big beehive hairstyle. Italian women are proud of their roots, and they carry themselves with heads held high. It's all about femininity.

Italians—they are the real divas!

# Get the Look

*Cream base foundation for matte finish. Loose powder.*

*Matte white eye shadow on the lids. Dark gray on the crease. Blend well.*

*Black thick liquid eyeliner, which was very popular in the 1960s, makes dramatic wings/extensions.*

*Black mascara and thick, longer-size fake eyelashes.*

*Dark eyebrows. I used matte, dark gray eye shadow.*

*Matte, light pink to nude lips.*

## PARIS LOOK

French beauty has a long history extending to before the French Revolution in 1789. Movie stars like Brigitte Bardot, Catherine Deneuve, and Jeanne Moreau created the modern images of classy French beauty.

This cinema look is all about bedroom eyes that have a hint of the '60s look, like Italians; the difference is that the French look is softer and "quieter."

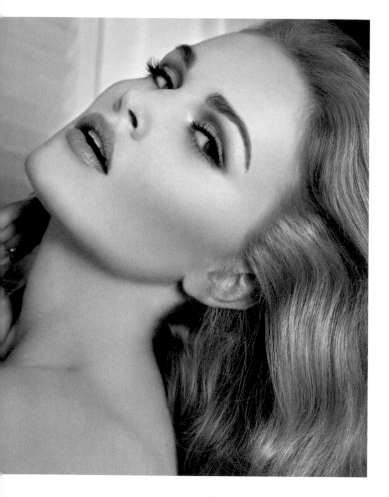

## Get the Look

*Cream foundation for more matte and satin finish. Matte face powder.*

*Light brown eye shadow on the lash line and crease. Blend well.*

*Dark brown liquid eyeliner.*

*Black mascara and black fake lashes (natural-length thicker '60s style).*

*Nude-color lips. Don't line the lips; just tap the lipstick on with the help of a lip brush.*

## STOCKHOLM LOOK

Nordic women love to wear bright colors in the summertime, when the sun never sets. Summertime is the time for celebration, and it is the only time of the year when makeup really shows on these Viking women. My inspiration was the '70s eye makeup, with a lot of black mascara and turquoise-blue eye shadow that was a popular look on Abba's lead singer, Agnetha Fältskog. The Scandinavian woman takes skin care seriously by taking facials regularly throughout the year. She also goes to a sauna at least once or twice a week to keep her skin clean and smooth.

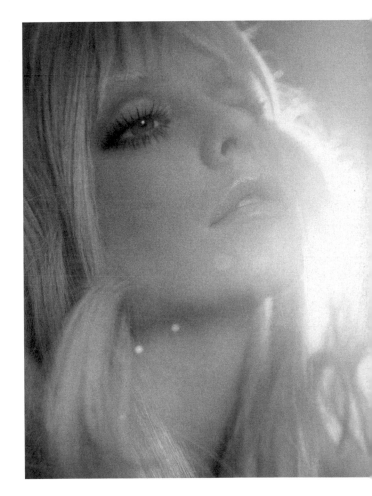

## *Get the Look*

*Lightest-tinted moisturizer,
no powder, to keep the skin dewy.*

*Eyes: blue-turquoise matte
eye shadow on the crease.
Blend it well.*

*Black mascara on the upper
and lower lashes.
Comb well.*

*Lips: clear gloss.*

*Blush: icy pink,
just to give color on the apples.*

## MADRID LOOK

Love, passion, fire, fight—those terms are strongly associated with Spanish-style beauty. It's all about those well-lined red bull's blood–colored lips and sharp black liner that looks like a bull-fighter's sword blade. The inspiration for this look was also Pedro Almodóvar's movie *Matador,* with all its passion.

# Get the Look

*Keep the face totally matte by using a cream foundation and loose powder.*

*Line the lips carefully with a deep red lip liner. Make sure the red is not too orange red—more like red wine or burgundy. Keep the lips matte.*

*Base the eyelids with ivory white matte eye shadow. This will make the eye makeup look simple and graphic along with the black liquid liner. Don't make the liner thick, as in the Italian look. Extend the liner with shorter wings.*

*Add false lashes to create more passionate drama.*

*The brows are filled with matte dark gray eye shadow.*

*The nails are red, sharp, and pointy as swords.*

## NEW YORK LOOK

American beauty is a celebration of varied skin colors. For many, true American beauty implies a fresh and natural look that radiates a positive and happy spirit. Extremely good nail and hair care as well as a beautiful smile are the most gorgeous elements of American beauty.

PHOTO: GITTE MELDGAARD/MODELS: CANDICE @ NOUS AND ANDRE @ VISION/HAIR: YIOTIS/NAILS: JENNA HIPP

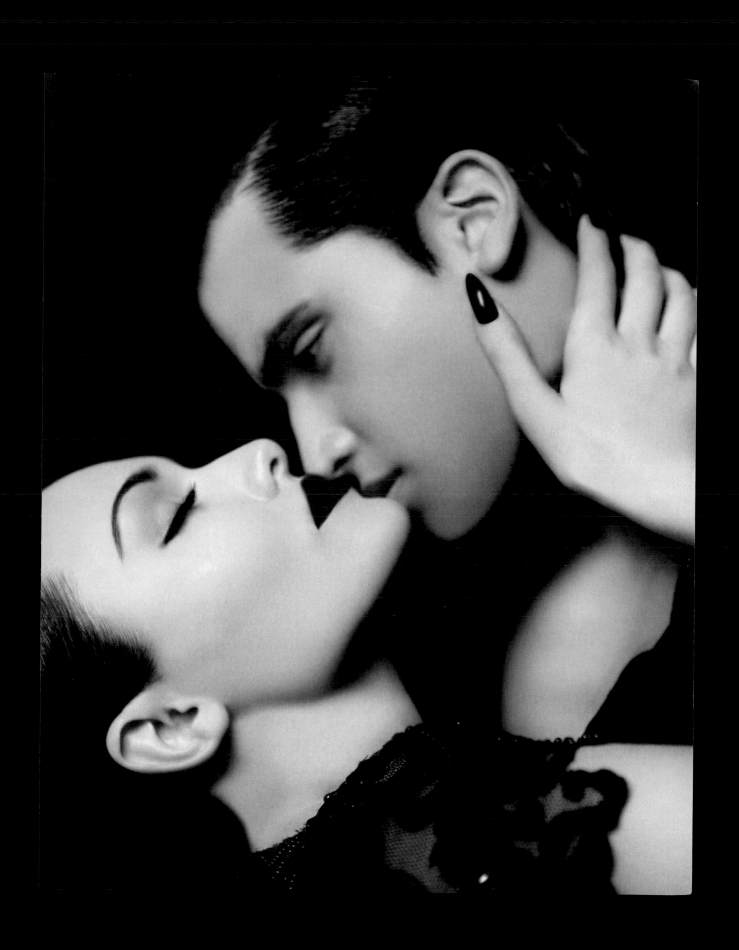

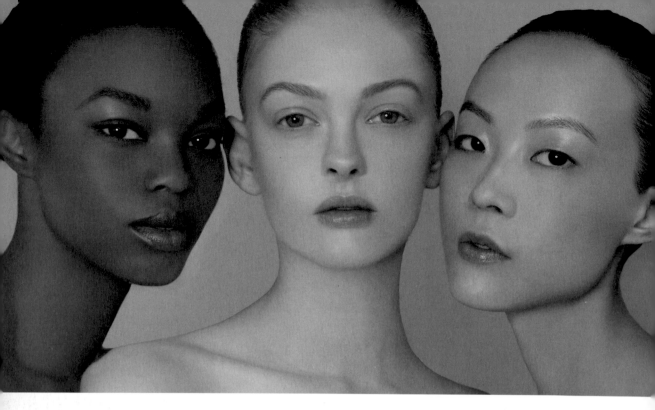

# Get the Look

*Use a tinted moisturizer and powder the face lightly.*

*Make the skin look very natural, as if you are not wearing any base.*

*Black mascara.*

*Use a little highlighter on the eyelids to give a beautiful sheen.*

*Tinted lip balm.*

*Keep the brows very natural but still beautifully groomed.*

PHOTO: GITTE MELDGAARD/MODELS: EUGENIA @ PHOTOGENICS,
DANI @ PHOTOGENICS, LESLIE @ FORD/HAIR: YIOTIS

# LONDON LOOK

The foggy and often rainy island's beauty is all about pale matte skin and deep red lips. The inspirations are Queen Elizabeth I, the fashion icon Grace Coddington, the rebel-punk London style that always dares to mix something new and vintage together and make it look right, and Vivienne Westwood's '90s fashion show makeups, which introduced clown-white faces and deep red lips.

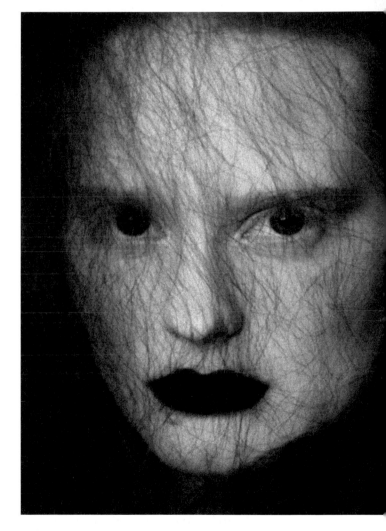

## Get the Look

*Skin: the most ivory cream foundation and lightest-color face powder. Keep it matte.*

*Eyes: nothing on the eyes.*

*Lips: the deepest red-wine color for the liner. Line the lips well and fill them with the liner.*

*Blush: add blush in the English Rose style on the apples of your cheeks.*

## TOKYO LOOK

Face whitening has played a big part in some Asian culture, and today face-whitening cosmetic products are one of the most sold items in Asia.

My Tokyo girl with a pale face and bold futuristic makeup represents the new Asian makeup generation. The Tokyo Look loves and dares to try new ways to express with makeup colors, a strong attitude, and high-tech style. Here comes the future!

## *Get the Look*

*Cream foundation: the lightest color.*

*Loose powder: the lightest color.*

*You can use neon colors or any other bright color choices on your lids.*
*I used yellow and green.*

*Bright fuchsia blush in shimmer.*
*Start the application from the temples and follow down to the apples.*
*Make it strong!*

*Nude lips keep this look together.*

*Also play with the nail polish—green, yellow, magenta, blue . . .*

PHOTO: GITTE MELDGAARD/MODEL: TEANI @ PHOTOGENICS/NAILS: JENNA HIPP/STYLING: HEIDI MEEK

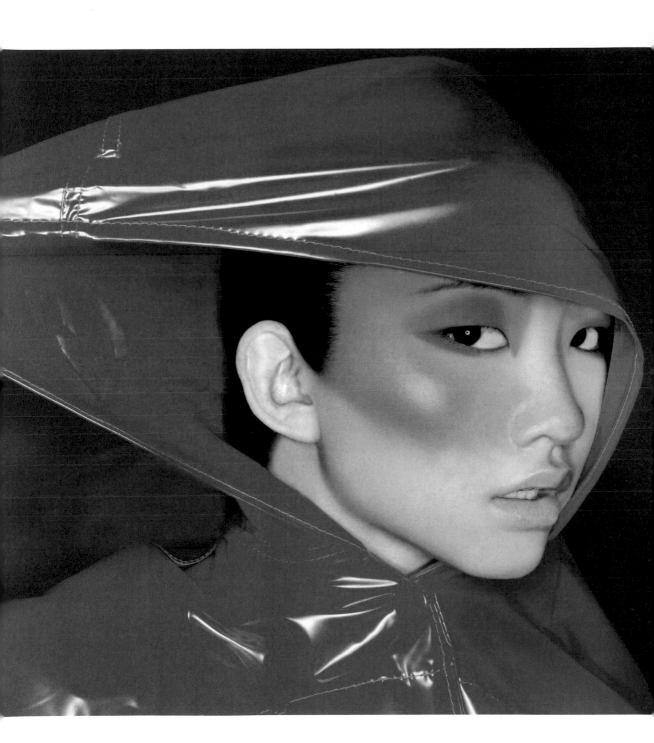

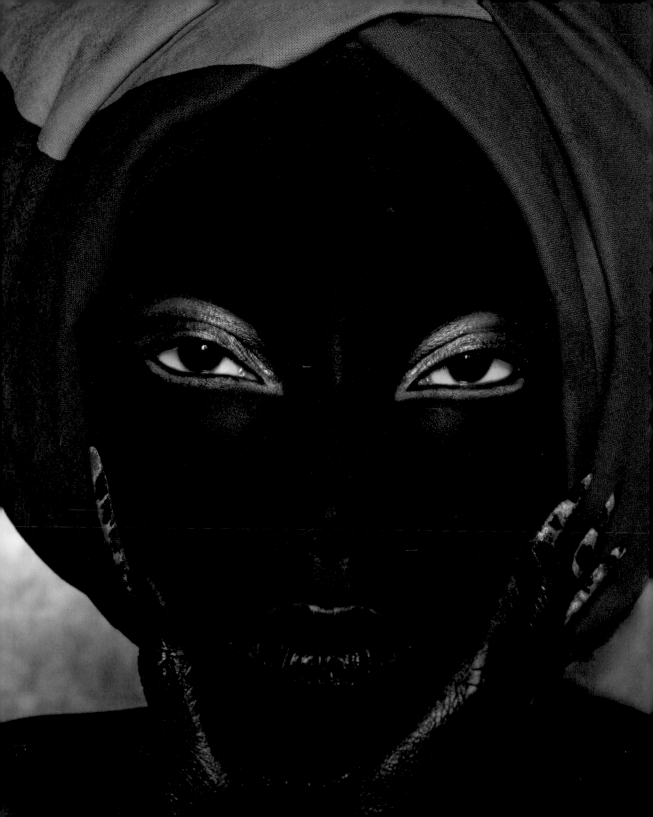

## NAIROBI LOOK

In my makeup, I wanted to create something very special and eye-catching that would create a beautiful message of African culture that is filled with colors and sounds, spirituality and pureness, as well the power of nature. I used gold supershimmer eye shadow in a powder format just around the eyes.

# Get the Look

*I didn't want Canise's skin to look matte, so I tapped a little bit of face oil on her skin to make it look more dewy.*
*When your skin is so dark, you just want to bring out that amazing color with some highlighting.*

*I applied gold shimmery eye shadow all around her amazing cat's eyes, which really came alive with this shimmer.*

*The nail artist Jenna Hipp made amazing high-fashion overlength fake nails to give a couture look.*

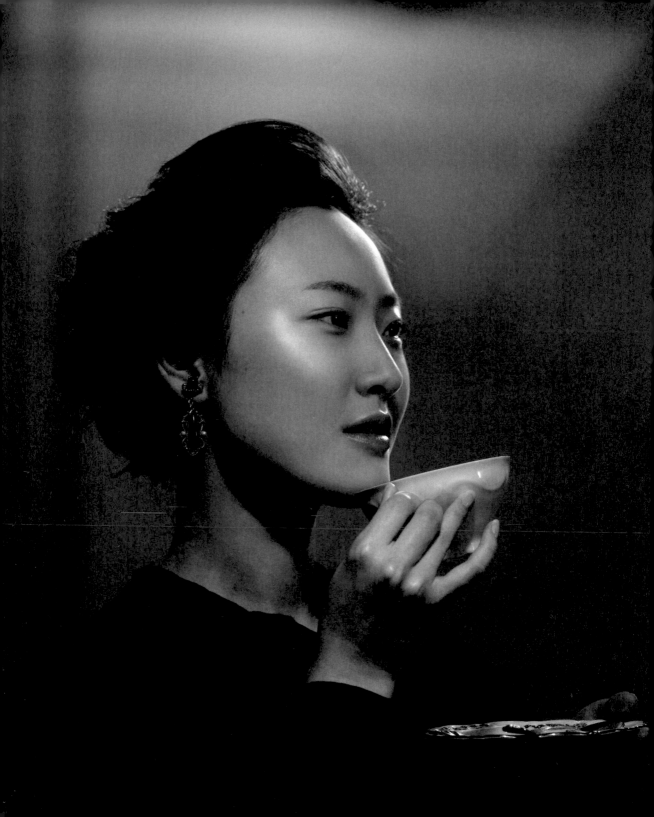

PHOTO: KURT ISWARIENKO/MODEL: KAREN @ FORD/HAIR: KEIKO HAMAGUCHI/NAILS: BETH FRICKE/PROPS: AMY HOLLAND

# 40 RETRO LOOKS

## (1900–1990s)

**Retro looks are very important in today's makeup creations. The 1920s were the first time since the ancient Egyptians that the unlimited use of cosmetics came to be universally accepted, both socially and morally. Every decade since has brought a totally new look in beauty. We professionals always get inspiration from the past. And then we mix the old ideas with today's modern vibes.**

## 1900–1920

At the beginning of the twentieth century, women wore very little makeup. Face powder was the most popular product, one that even the most conservative ladies found acceptable. The face was supposed to look pink or white, if possible, and women avoided going out in sunny weather. Or if they did, they put a little glycerine on the face, then passed a powder puff lightly over it, and finally covered the face with a cream-colored veil.

Another makeup product that came out was blush, in powder, pomade, and liquid formulas. In 1917, the first waterproof rouge saw daylight. The eyebrows at the beginning of the century were thick and well penciled with Chinese ink and rose water. The lips were natural or a light rose color. Rose water was used to give a light stain. The skin had a healthy glow, but the trend was to keep it pale.

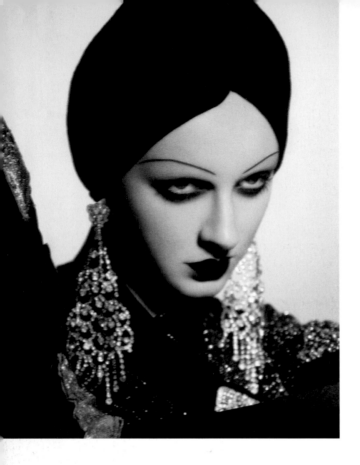

This makeup represents an old-Hollywood silent movie star look. It's very mysterious with dark eyes, thin penciled eyebrows, and small Cupid's-bow lips.

## Get the Look
### Silent Movie Queen

*Cream foundation or traditional pancake foundation to create the perfect satin and more-coverage finish.*

*Transparent loose powder.*

*The eye makeup is very theatrical, with the shape of "sad" eyes. Use only dark gray eye shadow (black looks too hard) to create this look. Make the eyes round. The eyebrows are thin and heavily drawn in a downhill shape. Cover your own brows with the help of a special brow wax (Kryolan makes a good one). Take a small amount of wax in the finger and press and pull the wax over the brows, making sure every single hair is totally covered. Cover the brows with pancake foundation and loose powder. Use light brown pencil to replace the shape of the brows on the top of the foundation (before powdering), so you can easily wipe off a wrong line and correct it. After powdering, it's easy to paint the brows with black liquid eyeliner.*

*Three coats of black mascara on the upper and lower lashes.*

*The lips are drawn very small, as a heart shape. Use deep red liner only.*

*Light pink blush in the middle of the cheeks to create a rounder face.*

## Late 1920s

The Jazz Age started in 1926 and lasted only three or four years, but it is the most memorable look of the '20s because of the flappers, the new rebelling young women who danced their nights out, cut their hair in the popular bob style, smoked cigarettes, and applied lipstick openly on the streets and in nightclubs. The fashion was all about shorter dresses (just under the knees) and the It Girls of the era were movie stars like Colleen Moore, Josephine Baker, Clara Bow, and Louise Brooks, who all had short bobs.

The makeup was still dark around the eyes but now also had options in green and blue eye shadows. The eyebrows were often plucked off to get the downward shape. Even though pale skin was still fashionable, the accidental sunburn of the designer Coco Chanel's face made the sun-kissed look extremely popular as well.

The lips were painted into a Cupid's-bow shape and a little thicker than in the early 1920s. New lipstick colors were raspberry and orange red.

## 1930s

After the flapper era, Wall Street crashed and a deep depression shook the world. But it didn't affect the use of cosmetics.

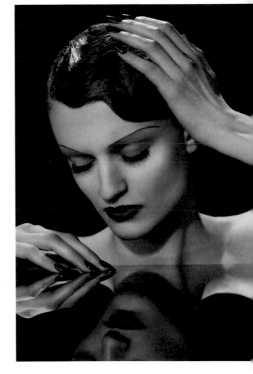

Cold creams, blushes, powders, and lipsticks sold well, and nail polish grew in popularity. Even in hard times, women wanted to look good. The 1930s look was more sophisticated and elegant than the overly theatrical look of the 1920s.

The 1930s are often called "The Hollywood Golden Era." The movies needed to provide entertainment for people during the Depression, and the glamorous silver screen divas gave women hope and a chance to forget their worries for a couple of hours by watching high-fashion silk-jersey gowns and fur coats on the big screen.

Makeup was simple and graphic, and hairdos followed with well-sculptured side- or middle-part finger waves. The look of this era was all about melancholy eyes and well-lined lips. Good examples are Hollywood royalty such as Greta Garbo (who was one of the rare stars to make it to the talkies after the silent era ended), Bette Davis, and Carole Lombard.

The eyebrows were often plucked very thin and drawn with the help of a dark brown or dark gray pencil. Good examples of '30s eyebrows are those of the movie stars Marlene Dietrich and Jean Harlow, whose superthin brows represent the highest fashion of the '30s look. The early '30s look was still influenced by the '20s small Cupid's-bow lip makeup, but in the late '30s the lip line was drawn all the way to the corners of the mouth.

## 1940s

The use of cosmetics decreased slightly during World War II because of shortages of the ingredients needed to produce them. The makeup was all about true red military lips, and the upper lip line was sometimes drawn slightly over the natural lip line to get the strong, almost bitchy lip look inspired by the leading Hollywood film divas. The eyebrows were thicker, and the shape was more arched, not round as in the '30s. The face was matte, with pancake makeup and loose powder. The look was cold and serious.

The beauty icons of the era were Lauren Bacall, Veronica Lake, and Greer Garson. Ingrid Bergman represented a more natural beauty. Betty Grable, Rita Hayworth, and Lana Turner were some of the movie stars whose pictures decorated the lockers of American soldiers overseas.

# Get the Look

*Concealer under the eyes and to cover any uneven areas on the face.*

*Cream foundation to give full coverage.*

*Transparent loose powder to keep the face matte.*

PHOTO: KURT ISWARIENKO/MODEL: PRISCILLA @ NOUS/HAIR: KEIKO HAMAGUCHI/PROPS: LISA LUPO

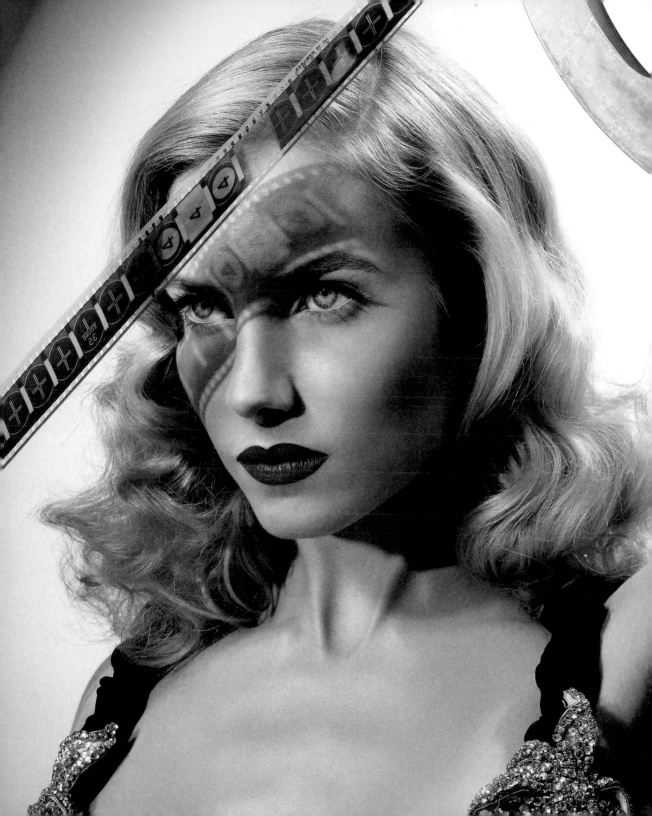

*Two eye shadows: ivory matte on the eyelids and light brown matte on the crease.*

*Just a hint of brown eye shadow to open up the eyes; no cat's-eye shape, just follow the crease of the eyes.*

*Black mascara and fake lashes.*

*White kohl inside the lids to open up the eyes.*

*Brows: matte eye shadow to give the strong '40s eyebrow style; thick brow and sharp arch.*

*Lips: lined with a warm red liner and filled with the liner as well. In the '40s women sometimes wore Vaseline over the lip makeup, especially in the movies, where actresses had to look superglamorous.*

*Blush: face contoured with a darker blush to achieve the hollow-face effect.*

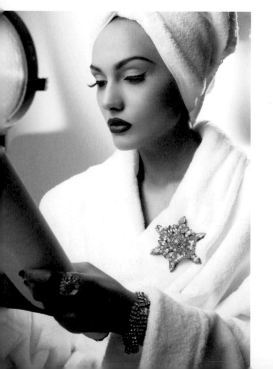

## 1950s

The winter of 1949–1950 saw a new beginning in Paris, a revolution in eye makeup: the doe-eyed look. Eyeliner was born. The makeup was fuller, with red lips, beautifully arched brows, orange-red lips, and well-lined eyes. Sales of eye makeup went wild on both sides of the Atlantic. Mascara, eye shadow, and liner were the top-selling items. New colors were used on the lids, such as light blue, turquoise, light gray, and green.

In the 1950s, the biggest fashion after the Dior look was rock 'n' roll, which became the new trend for youngsters all over the world. High ponytails and shorter "pixie" haircuts gave a more relaxing vibe for the superglam 1950s Hollywood look.

The new silver screen beauties of the time, such as Ava Gardner, Grace Kelly, and Elizabeth Taylor, gave Hollywood new class and glamor. And the stars Marilyn Monroe, Rosalind Russell, Kim Novak, and Anita Ekberg created a more erotic vibe for the era. The new teen idols were Sandra Dee and Annette Funicello.

# Get the Look

*Foundation: Max Factor Pan Cake was now a mainstream base product. It sold 10 million pieces a year.*

*Powder: loose yellow-based powder.*

*Eyes: white semimatte eye shadow all over the lids, up to the crease.*

*Black liquid eyeliner with extension wings. Black mascara and fake eye lashes no. 4, as on page 101.*

*Eyebrows: matte gray or light brown eye shadow. Make the eyebrows perfectly groomed, lined, and measured. The shape is more round, rather than hard and arched as in the '40s.*

*Lips: orange-red lip liner and the same color lipstick.*

## 1960s

There is not one way to describe 1960s makeup, because of its very different variations through the decade. The very early '60s look was sophisticated and gave a hint of what was coming up: the lips were lightened with light coral, apricot, sand, and cinnamon lipstick. Eye shadow was a little bit darker, with matte browns and grays. The shadow was now also applied to the lower lash line, but still very light-handed.

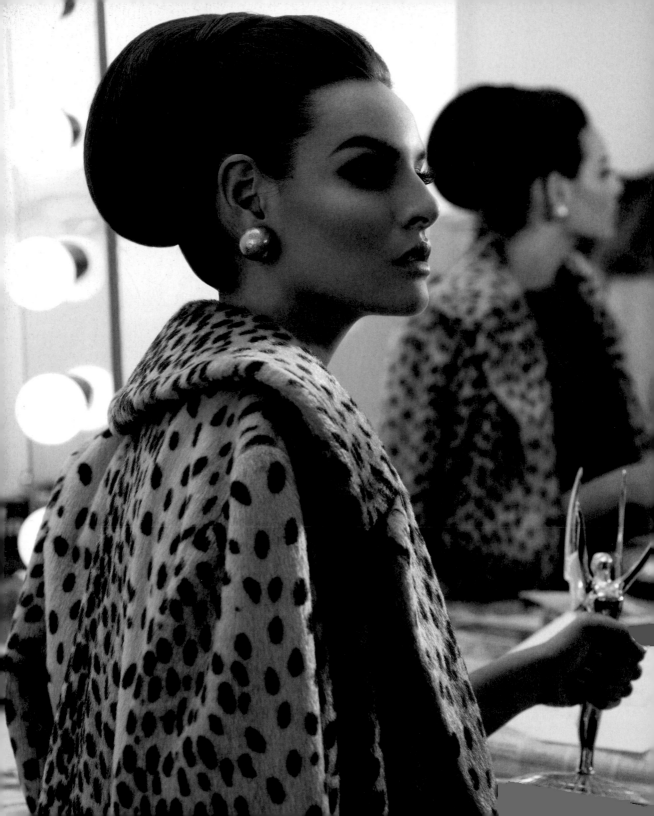

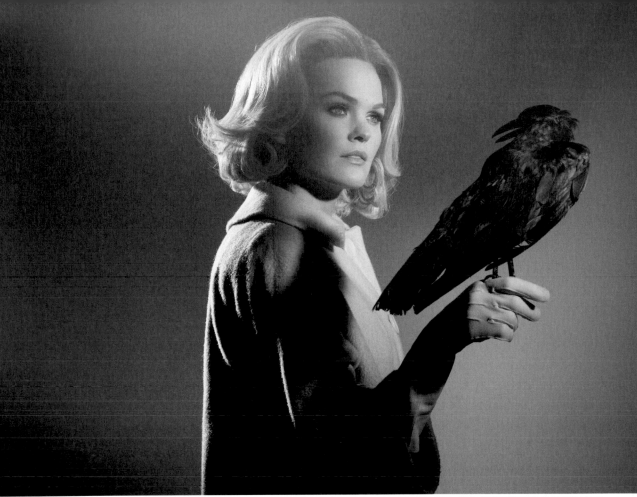

PHOTO: KURT ISWARIENKO/MODEL: SUNNY MABREY/HAIR: ROB TALTY/PROPS: AMY HOLLAND

PHOTO: KURT ISWARIENKO/MODEL: ANNE @ INDUSTRY/
HAIR: KEIKO HAMAGUCHI/NAILS: BETH FRICKE

Liquid eyeliner was slightly thicker, and false eyelashes were widely used. Eyebrows were darker and thicker, and the shape was more graphic than in the '50s.

The look I created got its inspiration from Alfred Hitchcock's movie *The Birds* (1963) and its leading lady, Tippi Hedren, whose look represents the more sophisticated and elegant American look of the early 1960s.

The actress Sunny Mabrey has the perfect face for this makeup as a retro star. This typical mid-1960s glamorous evening look is all about the eyes. Darker matte brown eye shadow was applied very strongly on the upper and lower lids, creating the elegant look of the 1960s. The shape of the shadow is triangular.

Thick fake eyelashes were used on the upper lashes to give the eyes depth,

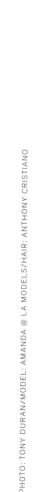

and bottom fake lashes to opened the eyes even more. Liquid black eyeliner was the main makeup product in the mid-1960s.

The brows are strong and graphic. The arch is made very graphic and strong. The lips are a pale salmon color (I used a lip liner to color the lips and kept the lines very soft and natural).

Contouring was done with darker sand-color blush. The nails are light pink, sand, or ivory colors. White inside liner was now used to open up the eyes, especially for evening looks. Hollywood stars such as Natalie Wood, Shirley MacLaine, Faye Dunaway, Jane Fonda, Barbra Streisand, and Mia Farrow were the faces of the new generation of the cinema. The European stars Sophia Loren, Ursula Andress, and Brigitte Bardot were also noticed by the American audience, thanks to their amazing '60s sexy siren looks. Diana Ross provided the superglam look for music, and Donyale Luna was the first African-American supermodel to appear on the covers of fashion magazines.

## Veruschka

This look got its inspiration from Paco Rabanne fashion and the German supermodel Veruschka. It was all about black liner in a triangular frame and white eye shadow and eye pencil. The '60s eye makeup also was very futuristic, and silver, gold, and bronze were used a lot, especially in 1967 and after.

## Twiggy

The London look was about the Mary Quant fashion, which included a Vidal Sassoon haircut, a new graphic and modern style that even today looks fresh and super-modern. The Mod look also came from London. It was for new modern women who

PHOTO: TONY DURAN/MODEL: AMANDA @ LA MODELS/HAIR: ANTHONY CRISTIANO

cut their as hair graphic round-shaped bobs and had dark matte eye makeup and pale lips. The fashion model Twiggy was the "It Girl" with her wide-open eyes, spidery lashes, and light lips. The Brits set the trends, and the rest of the world followed.

The most creative, extreme, and unique makeup was worn by Peggy Moffitt, the model and muse of the Austrian-born fashion designer Rudi Gernreich. Her alien-looking big eye makeup is iconic.

## 1970s

The 1970s were very interesting in the history of makeup.

Hippie culture was still going strong in the early '70s, and it inspired more creativity in fashion and makeup.

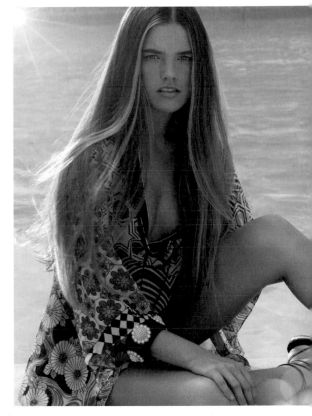

Some women were using poster paints around the eyes and watercolors on the face, or painting rainbows above their eyes. The eyebrows were also bleached for a unique look, and the forehead was painted in a triangle shape with pink, green, and yellow eye shadows. This look was the wild version of the '70s and was unique rather than conventionally beautiful.

But in the early '70s there was also a totally opposite, more down-to-earth look that went hand in hand with the ideology of a natural, healthy lifestyle. Natural skin care ingredients such as papaya, cucumber, avocado, sesame seeds, and almonds were used again, as they had been thousands of years before, and new makeup products were developed. Women practiced yoga, meditation, and self-hypnosis. In the mid- and late '70s, makeup went wild again, with new colors and ways to enhance it. Fashion designers such as Halston, Yves Saint Laurent, Kenzo Takada, and Sonia Rykiel created the frames for makeup and hairstyles. Disco music was

PHOTO: DANIELA FEDERICI/MODEL: AMANDA @ IMG/HAIR: DAMIAN MONZILLO/PUBLISHED AT HAMPTONS

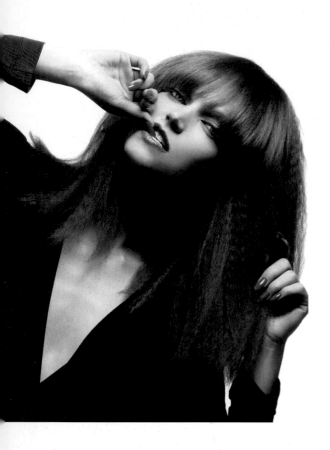

born and clubbing gave a new attitude for fashion and beauty. New York's nightclub Studio 54 was the it place to go partying if you were rich and famous.

Beauty icons of the '70s included Lauren Hutton, Beverly Johnson, Farrah Fawcett, Jerry Hall, Margaux Hemingway, Bianca Jagger, Jessica Lange, and the androgynous David Bowie.

The opposite of fancy and fashionable clubbing was punk, which gave a new, radical way of seeing the future. Punks wore dark cat-eye makeups and black or red lips, and piercing was a popular body art. Nails were painted black.

This late-'70s makeup is inspired by the French fashion designer Sonia Rykiel, punk, and Studio 54.

The overall look is very strong, with long, orange-red nails that emphasize the strong attitude that carried all the way through to the early 1980s. The look also uses black inside kohl, orange-red lip gloss, and a strong orange blush applied from the temples down to the apples of the cheeks in an L-shape. The skin was semimatte, and eye shadows were shimmery.

## 1980s

The fast-moving '80s were an era of extravagance: clothes, hair, makeup, and a yuppie lifestyle that you had to be able afford—or pretend to. Beauty got its inspiration from movies and TV series such as *American Gigolo*, *Flashdance*, and *Dynasty*. MTV was the biggest trendsetter, with new stars such as Cyndi Lauper, Madonna, Debbie Harry of Blondie, Jody Watley, and Whitney Houston.

The new generation of Hollywood stars included Nastassia Kinski, Rebecca

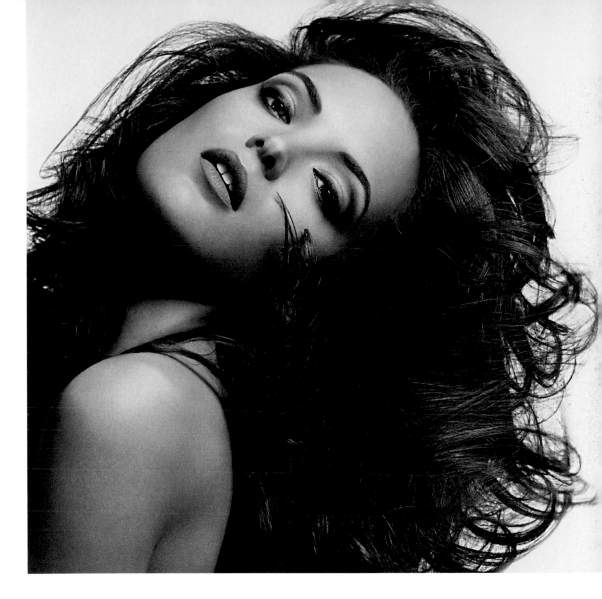

De Mornay, Julia Roberts, Kelly McGillis, Tom Cruise, Richard Gere, and Rob Lowe. New faces such as Cindy Crawford, Paulina Porizkova, Iman, Yasmin Le Bon, and Christy Turlington dominated the fashion and beauty industries.

Makeup was strong, with a futuristic vibe. The early-'80s look was still influenced by punk, with strong black kohl eye makeup and red matte lips. The mid-'80s featured neon makeup colors. Eyebrows were shaped strong and graphic. Foundation was used for full coverage, and makeup was kept as matte as possible.

# Get the Look

*This supermodel look I created is a typical '80s editorial makeup that was seen in many international fashion magazines. The makeup is strong in both the eyes and the lips.*

*Make the eyes extended "cat's eyes" and use two to three coats of mascara. Black kohl inside the eyes, just as in the late-'70s makeup, gives that strong attitude.*

*The lips are fuchsia, and I used a lip liner to create the color.*

## 1990s

The early '90s were still all about big shoulder pads, big hair, and strong makeup, but in 1993 everything changed, when grunge revolutionized the fashion world. It was time to lie back, relax, and breathe again after many years of strong makeup, glitter, and a too-ambitious lifestyle and snobbish attitude. Seattle became the city of grunge, launching such bands as Nirvana (its lead singer, Kurt Cobain, was the real trendsetter of the grunge style) and Soundgarden. The fashion world quickly followed this new style, and soon Kate Moss was hired by Calvin Klein to bring a more relaxed and new-generation vibe its advertising.

Fashion became more creative and modern, thanks to more edgy designers such as Ann Demeulemeester, Comme des Garçons, Yohji Yamamoto, Helmut Lang, Marc Jacobs, Dries Van Noten, and Alexander McQueen, to name a few of the most influential designers of the era.

Hip-hop and techno music became popular worldwide.

New faces freshened the catwalks and fashion magazines: Kristen McMenamy (whose trademarks were shaved eyebrows and a short black '20s-style black bob) and the Canadian model Eve (with her shaved and tattooed head) complemented the bigger beauties of that era: Linda Evangelista, Naomi Campbell, Tatiana Patitz, and Shalom Harlow, to name a few.

Grunge makeup was androgynous. Black kohl and a pencil liner were applied together on the upper and lower lids, then smudged with the fingers, with the help

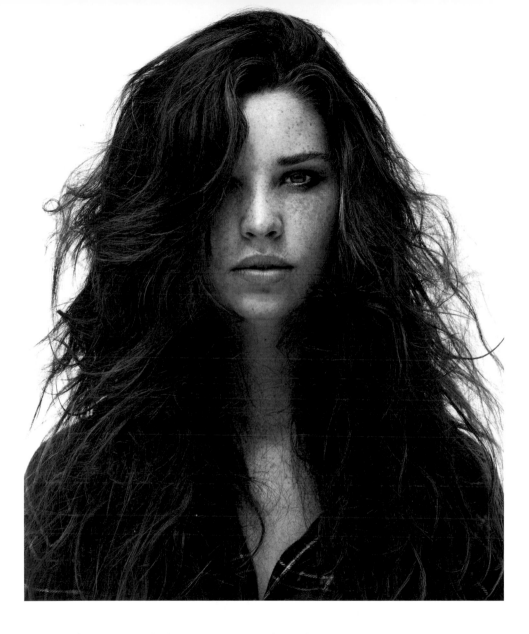

PHOTO: KURT ISWARIENKO/MODEL: MORGAN @ FORD/HAIR: ROB TALTY

of a bit of Vaseline, which gave a sexy and trendy "heroin" look. Male rockers loved the look as well.

The skin was bare, with no makeup. Lips were sometimes painted deep gothic red or even black, with no eye makeup. Face and body piercings made a big comeback.

Hollywood's new megastars were Alicia Silverstone, Winona Ryder, Sherilyn Fenn, Nicole Kidman, and Angelina Jolie.

# 41 COSMETICS CARE

**When did you last take an inventory of all your cosmetics? Maybe there are some face creams that you bought two years ago but haven't even opened yet, and you wonder if can you still use them. How about that beloved red lipstick that you have saved for five years? What about that loose powder that you totally forgot to use? Here are some helpful answers for your inventory questions from an expert who has worked in the cosmetics industry since 1964.**

**Marita Tabermann Coccaro,** *cosmetics developer and CEO of TaberCo*

### *How do I know when skin care products, like my creams and toners, are too old and I can't use them anymore?*

Check the product's shelf life. The label indicates the product's last use date, but it's no more than 18 to 24 months from the second you open them. If you have a face cream that you bought two years ago but haven't opened, don't use it. Throw it away! Two years (24 months) is the limit. Today products have fewer preservatives, which means a shorter shelf life. European products always indicate for how many months you can use the product after you open the package. If there isn't any shelf life info, you can always call the cosmetics company and ask.

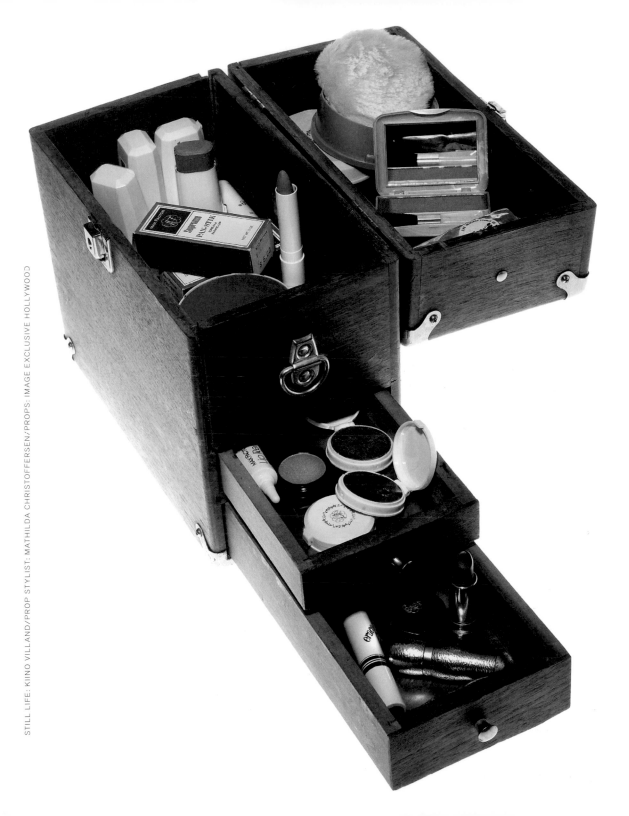

### How long can I use my foundation before it gets old?

One year. Even if you think that you can use it after a year, you must throw it away because of the bacteria. You may think you can use it longer, but after a year you'll realize that you have used only half of the product. Always buy a 30-milliliter or smaller container.

### How long can I use my concealers?

One year.

### Do powders get old or develop harmful bacteria?

Loose powder is okay to use for two years. The problem is the powder puff; you apply the puff to your face and put it back into the powder. It collects bacteria and oils from your skin and transfers them to the powder. You must wash your powder puffs in warm water and soap once a week to keep them free of oils, dirt, and bacteria. And never throw your powder puff into your makeup purse after you use it. Keep it in a small ziplock plastic bag, so it stays more hygienic.

### Do lipsticks and lip glosses get old or develop harmful bacteria?

Lipsticks last the longest because they don't have a base for bacterias (they are wax-based). But after three years, throw them away. Lip gloss: one year—out.

### How about eye pencils and lip pencils?

Three years. You must always remember to put the cap on the pencil, otherwise it will dry out. And sharpen it as well, to reveal the clean surface!

### Do powder-format eye shadows and blushes get old?

Everything depends on how hygienic you are with your brushes and the application. You must wash your brushes often. We professionals do so every day, at least once or twice a day, so you should do so at least twice week to avoid bacteria building up on the blush or eye shadows. Three years, again, is a good time to change eye shadows or blushes. Even if you don't think they look old, you never know how many bacteria have built up on the top layer of the product.

### Is it true I can use a tube of mascara for only two months?

Yes. Mascara—two months, period. When you pump oxygen into the tube, bacteria from the air go into the mascara.

### What is the best storage place for creams and other skin care products?

A bathroom cabinet that is dark and cool. You can even store some items, such as eye-area cream and gel, in your refrigerator. They feel better on your skin when they are cooler. All products such as face toners that contain water as their first ingredient store very well in the refrigerator.

# 42 MEN AND COSMETICS

**Men's cosmetics today are more than just a soap bar, a razor, and cologne. In the 1960s, cosmetics companies started to develop more men's skin care and grooming products, and the market really exploded by the mid-'80s. Today there are more than enough men's skin care lines out there to make it all quite confusing. How do you choose the day cream that suits you? Before anything else, determine what your skin type is: dry, combination, or oily.**

Depending on your skin type, you will choose your skin care routine from A.M. to P.M. Refer to chapter 1, "Facial Care," which includes information from the skin care guru Ole Henriksen. I fought with my own skin starting in my teens until I hit 28. My skin used to be very dry and sensitive (it's now combination but still sensitive). I had to moisturize my skin more than anyone could ever imagine. Coming from northern Europe, the cold winter was really my enemy. I learned from my very early years to save my skin using special treatments that my mother taught me. (My mother was a skin-obsessed pharmacist who took wonderful care of me and my skin.) One of them was evening primrose oil; I took it for two years, and my skin healed a lot. I also opened the capsules and applied it directly to my skin before a sauna and under my day cream. My mother taught me that changing face creams every couple of months is refreshing for the skin, so every two to three weeks I get a new face cream. It always feels so great and new on my skin. (I use only hypoallergenic face oils, gel-lotions, and creams as well as body creams.)

Skin care has always been very important to me, and I tell my male clients about the importance of a proper skin care program.

TODAY'S GROOMING IS MORE RELAXED AND EVEN BOHEMIAN, BUT YOU STILL WANT TO LOOK WELL PUT TOGETHER: SKIN, HAIR, AND NAIL CARE IS AS IMPORTANT AS YOUR DAILY NUTRITION AND EXERCISE. IT'S AS MUCH ABOUT FEELING GOOD AS LOOKING GOOD.

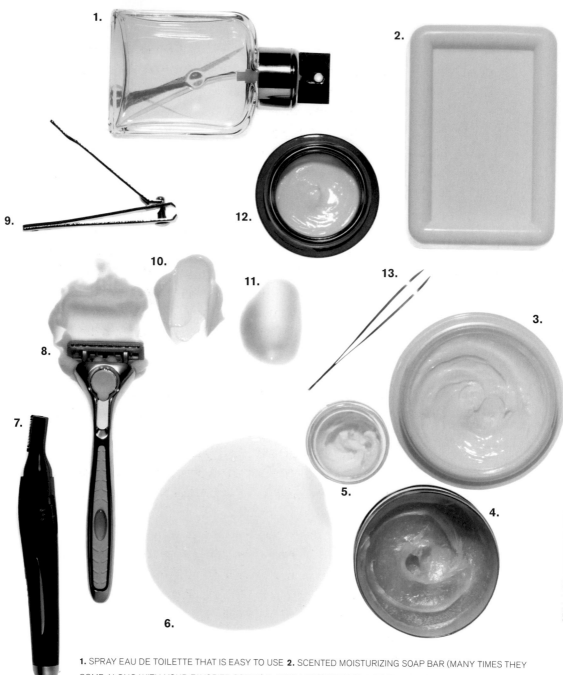

1. SPRAY EAU DE TOILETTE THAT IS EASY TO USE 2. SCENTED MOISTURIZING SOAP BAR (MANY TIMES THEY COME ALONG WITH YOUR FAVORITE SCENT) 3. BODY MOISTURIZER 4. HAIR WAX FOR SHORT HAIRSTYLING 5. EYE-AREA CREAM FOR: MORNING AND EVENING 6. FACIAL WASH 7. A SMALL FACIAL HAIR TRIMMER TO KEEP THE NOSE AND EARS FREE OF HAIR 8. RAZOR AND SHAVING FOAM/GEL 9. NAIL CLIPPERS 10. MICRODERMABRASION SCRUB: USE ONE TO FOUR TIMES A WEEK, DEPENDING ON YOUR SKIN TYPE 11. LIP BALM 12. FACE CREAM FOR MORNING AND EVENING 13. TWEEZERS TO KEEP THE BROWS CLEAN LOOKING

**SHAVING:** If you like a clean look, you might have to shave three to seven times a week. Sometimes you might even need to shave twice a day. Use a shaving gel/foam instead of a soap bar. Why? Shaving foams/gels enable the razor to glide smoothly and more safely. Many shaving products have skin care benefits such as aloe and jojoba oil, which aid the skin and prevent irritation. Soap tends to get stuck between the blades and turns shaving into an unpleasant experience by slowing down shaving time and increasing the chance of breaking the skin.

**CLEANSING:** Wash your face every morning and evening with a facial wash. Use a gel or foam formulation for combination or oily skin, cream wash for dry skin. When you wash your face, the pores will be cleansed and you'll avoid clogs that will become black- or whiteheads. Finish cleansing with your skin-type toner. I like spray toners because they're easy to use and I really get that fresh feel by spraying the product on my face, especially in the morning. By keeping your face clean, you'll look and feel good!

**AFTERSHAVE:** This is very old school. Men used to apply a special aftershave lotion right after shaving that had a very masculine smell. What this actually did was more drying than really soothing and calming to the skin. I don't like aftershave products because they have a strong scent and I want to have the freedom to choose my own scent, and often my own favorite is completely opposite from what the aftershave product can offer. Scent is very personal.

**MOISTURIZING:** Skin care products are the new aftershave products; they calm and soothe the skin right after shaving. I love spray toners; which calm my skin, tighten the pores, and prepare my skin for moisturizer. I moisturize daily with a product containing SPF 15. If you have oily skin, use an oil-free moisturizing product. I personally like day creams with sun protectors, because I don't need to use two creams on top of each other. One face cream and I am ready to go. Eye-area gel/cream is a must for men as well. And keep lip balm with you at all times; nothing is more unattractive than dry, chapped lips!

**PROTECTING:** If you are vacationing near the water or snow, you need a higher SPF number than your 15 SPF day cream provides. Use at least SPF 30. Remember aftersun lotions or aloe vera gel for soothing and calming the skin, especially if you are spending more than three hours under direct sun each day. If your skin is burned, you can apply a 0.1% cortisone cream to the burned areas. Aloe vera gel also soothes burned skin.

**EXTRA CARE:** Exfoliate one to four times a week, depending on your skin type. If you have dry skin, do so once a week; for combination skin, do so on the oily areas two to three times a week; for oily skin, four times a week. This will wash off dead cells and make the skin softer and more even. I always exfoliate before shaving; the skin and hair become softer, my shaving is easier and smoother, and I never suffer from irritation (I exfoliate in the shower, which softens my skin with the steam). A facial mask is a great way to nurture the skin. Use a hydrating mask for dry skin and a clay mask for oilier areas. Calming and soothing masks are also great after shaving, if you have time. If you feel you are developing a pimple, use a blemish-attack product. It will work!

## MEN AND MAKEUP

Men don't usually think about using makeup on a daily basis, except for those who like to wear makeup or are actors or rock stars. But a little makeup can freshen up tired-looking eyes and even out skin tone. Gel-formula tinted moisturizer is a good option because the formulation is ultrathin and blends perfectly. Concealer can make your dark circles disappear. Just tap it under your eyes. Blotting paper will keep your oily skin matte. Lip balm is a must. Keep some with you at all times.

### I have acne. How should I shave?

First of all, always use a new, clean razor. If your razor blade is clogged with your old dry skin and hair and dirt, the blade won't glide over your skin smoothly and might break your skin on the areas where you have pimples. And then it is easy for bacteria to get inside the skin and infect it. So my first advice is: be very hygienic.

Then use an ultrasensitive shaving foam and let the razor do the work, not you—meaning be light-handed. Right after shaving, use cold water to rinse the foam off your face. (This will alleviate possible irritation and close the pores). Dab (don't rub) the skin dry with a clean towel, and use skin care products. Toner and oil-free moisturizer (SPF 15) will calm and soothe the skin. Also use a blemish-attack product to dry out any blemishes.

If you have a serious acne, you should always see a dermatologist and get medication as well as special skin care products to kill the bacteria and heal your skin. But remember that as much as you take good care of your acne with skin care products, your daily diet must include enough fiber, zinc, and raw foods, and you must avoid junk food, alcohol, tobacco, and processed foods in general. Be strict, and in time you will see the difference.

### How do I shave my head?

If your hairline is high and your hair is thin, shaving your hair off completely is an option. Nowadays this look is totally "in" and looks really cool. If you do have hair and want to have the bald look, you must use a clipper to get the hair as short as possible before shaving (clippers usually come with eight or nine different comb attachments). Use no. 1–2 to clip the hair shortest.

Take a shower. Keep the water running on your head for at least couple of minutes to soften the skin and hair. Use shaving gel or foam and a high-quality razor. Start shaving from front to back, and then go from side to side. A hand mirror is very practical for seeing the back of your head. Use your daily moisturizer on your head after shaving to moisten the skin and avoid developing redness or rashes.

### I have razor bumps and ingrown hair. What can I do?

How often do you shave? Shaving often to keep the hair short is the secret to not having bumps: when hair is always short, it can't grow back inside the skin surface. If you have an ingrown hair, ask your dermatologist to open the skin and pull the hair out.

### Are facials common for men?

Absolutely, yes! The new generation is more and more into skin care. Good skin is happy skin!

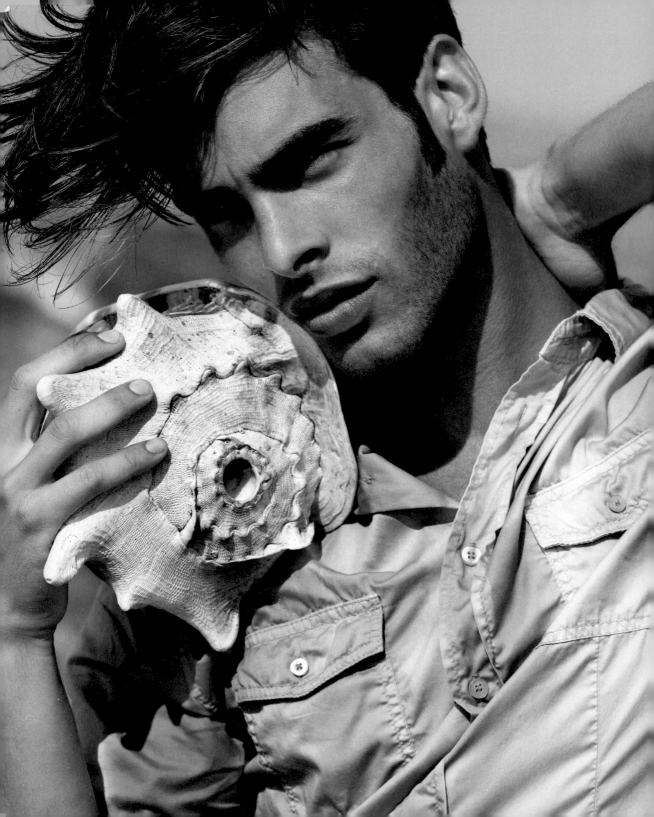

### What about mani-pedicures?

Pedicures are more popular than manicures for men. Every man should have a pedicure done once a month, or at least in the summer, when you will be wearing sandals. Why not choose a hair salon with pedicure services? I'm sure your loved one will be happy to see you with clean feet and toenails. You should also try a manicure once. See and feel the difference.

### Is waxing common in men?

Absolutely. Men get their chest, back, legs, and arms waxed, just as women do (well, less the chest and back!).

### How about eyebrows?

Read what the eyebrow specialist Gina says about men's eyebrows on page 73.

### What are good styles for a beard? How do I know which one will suit me?

There are so many different styles: goatee, sideburns, chinstrap, royale, circle beard, Fu Manchu, pencil mustache, soul patch, and full beard, just to name a few. It depends on your lifestyle, profession, and personal style; all of these elements give an idea of which style of beard or mustache you should choose. Your face shape is also important when choosing the most flattering facial hairstyle: for example, a round face looks best with a goatee, which will give the face more length; avoid sideburns or a full beard because they give too much roundness. The best way to get your most flattering beard is to see a hairstylist or barber who specializes in different styles of beards.

Use an electric trimmer and scissors or a clipper to trim your beard.

### What are the biggest beauty crimes for men?

- Dyeing gray hair but keeping the gray beard: always dye the beard as well to get a more natural result. If possible, use a professional colorist to do the job to avoid any surprises (too dark, red, or yellow).
- Allowing hair in the ears and nose to grow. Please trim it.
- Too-thick eyebrows in the middle make your eyes look too close together.

# 43 BODY MAKEUP

**Any time you will be wearing an evening gown that shows your décolleté and/or arms and legs, you should consider using body makeup—at least a good, thicker-formula body lotion. Why? Many times the color and texture of the body skin look a little bit different than your made-up face. It doesn't matter how perfect your foundation is compared to your neckline, but your décolleté might be sunburned, your legs might have a blue mark, or you might want to cover a birthmark on your back or smooth a scar on your hand. Your body skin might also look too ashy, pink, or pale compared to your face. It's time for body makeup.**

1.  **For blue marks,** see-through veins, birthmarks, sunburn, and other problems, use a high-pigment cream base: Joe Blasco, Ben Nye, Kryolan, or Cinema Secrets, which are very well known brands used by movie and theater makeup artists. They make really good products that work well. You apply the makeup only on the area you need to cover and blend it well. You don't need to powder, but if you have quite oily skin, a light powdering will keep the makeup from running. A more covering concealer does the same job if the area you need to cover is small. For bigger areas I prefer to use the high-pigment cream foundation. And make sure the shade blends perfectly with your own skin.

2.  **For too-ashy skin:** A thicker-formula body lotion will take care of this problem. It moisturizes the skin and gives it a beautiful glow. Two of my

favorites are Kiehl's Crème de Corps and Guerlain's Super Aqua Body Serum, which keep the skin moist and beautifully, naturally glowing for a long time.

### 3.  For too-pink, yellow, or pale skin:

You need a light-formula body makeup that covers naturally and gives the skin a dewy look. For skin that is too pale and pink, I prefer to use a little more yellow-based body makeup—but just a hint, because too much yellow starts to look too dark and dirty. If the skin is very pink, use a green-based color-correcting primer that will neutralize the pink of the skin. Take just a little product on the palms of your hands and apply it directly to the skin. Then apply the body makeup on top of that.

### 4.  Body bronzers are

terrific for medium and dark skin tones because they look natural and give the skin a beautiful sheen and glow. My favorite is a cream bronzer that I apply with my fingers, just like applying a body cream. Oil-based bronzers are too messy. Aerosol body bronzers are fine; they are fast to apply and do a good job. Just make sure not to choose too orange a color. Always test the product in natural light.

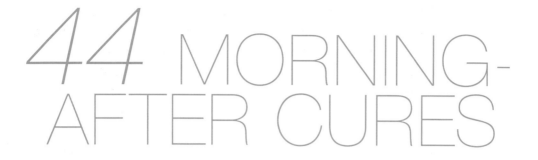

# 44 MORNING-AFTER CURES

We love nightlife but often pay for its pleasures with poor looks the day after. There are preventive measures and after-the-fact cures. The most important thing is to drink plenty of water on your night out. Remember this: after each alcoholic drink, have a big glass of water to hydrate your body. Right before you go to bed, maybe have a little snack to balance the salt and sugar levels of your body to avoid a headache—and drink some more water!

## IN THE MORNING

**5 Minutes:** Drink a big glass of water and take a warm shower. A lemon-citrus flavor shower/body wash lifts the mind and wakes you up. Exfoliate your face to wake it up (this enhances blood circulation and brings your face back to life!). You can do this in the shower. Dab your body dry and add a citrus-lemon body cream to moisturize your body. Spray a toner on your face to minimize the pores and prepare for the eye cream and serum. If your skin is very dry, you might need a nourishing day cream on top of the serum. Serum tightens the skin and gives it a minilift. It really freshens the face. You can massage the serum on your face to relax your facial muscles. If you have red eyes, remember eye drops.

**10 Minutes:** Not much time, but here we go: Use a concealer to cover up any red/uneven areas on your face. Tinted moisturizer really helps because it looks the most natural. If you have redness on your face, use a green-toned color-correcting primer under the tinted moisturizer. It magically washes most of the redness from your face. (For serious redness, use 0.1% cortisone cream.) For dark circles, use a light-reflecting pencil on top of the tinted moisturizer and blend it well.

Use neutral-tone makeup colors. Bright colors will make your tired face look even scarier. Keep your eye makeup natural: just matte shadow and mascara (remember to curl your lashes if you have straight ones—this really wakes up your eyes).

Blush is your best friend today. As always, blush will give your face warmth and life. Keep your lips natural. Line the lips with your usual color of liner and add a little bit of bright peach, nude, or icy pink lipstick. Add a little gloss to the center of the lips to get a fresher feel.

And now eat your breakfast and have a double espresso—and you are ready to face the day!

## Ole Henriksen: Rx for Puffy Eyes and Tired Skin

*Puffy eyes and bags are generally created by one of four causes: a diet high in salty foods; an overdose of alcohol, including wine; an allergic reaction to makeup or an eye cream; or crying. The best antidote for puffy eyes is to grate a cucumber and wrap the finely grated cucumber in cheesecloth to create a long, broad eye pad that will cover both eyes. This trick of creating a "sushi roll," if you will, prevents the paste from running all over the place, while allowing the vitamins and enzymes to release through the thin cloth. At my spa in West Hollywood, every complexion treatment includes the grated-cucumber eye treatment, and celebrities such as Charlize Theron, Renée Zellweger, and Ellen DeGeneres swear by this depuffing eye treatment. My Ultimate Lift Eye Gel is infused with a high concentration of cucumber extract for the same purpose.*

*Fill your bathroom sink one-third full of cold water and add a trayful of ice cubes. Drench a terry facecloth in the icy water, lay it across your face, and hold it firmly in place for one minute. Repeat at least five times. Your skin will be oxygenated and come to life in a matter of minutes. Follow with a facial mist. Stretching is another way to get circulation going to all your bodily extremities, so don't forget to do daily stretching excercises.*

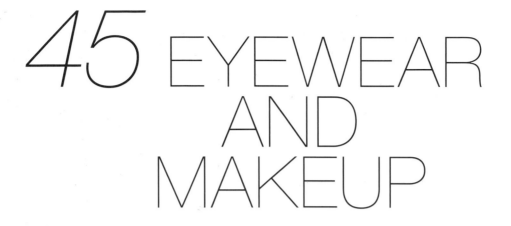

# 45 EYEWEAR AND MAKEUP

**Today's eyewear is an important accessory, like your your handbag, scarf, and shoes. You want to match it with your lifestyle, hair color, skin tone, and overall style. Sometimes you just want to buy a pair of cool-looking glasses even if you don't need any vision lenses. It's a myth that you should wear more eye makeup while wearing glasses. Maybe that was true in the '80s, when all beauty magazines advised wearing a lot of eye shadow to make your eyes pop. Today, keep it simple. Otherwise you will resemble the fabulous Dame Edna Everage, in all her glory (and we do love her).**

The design of the frames is very important: they must sit perfectly on your face. Your facial shape is once again important when choosing eyewear. What looks great on your best friend might not suit you at all because your facial shape is totally different; round-shaped eyewear, for example, might look great on an oval face, but it doesn't look the best on a round face. Then you might want to try narrower and longer frames. The material is also important: Do you want metallic or plastic frames? Transparent, brown, black, red, metallic, or maybe multicolored? All these elements will affect the way you do your makeup. If you have strong Japanese-design red plastic frames, you won't necessarily want to wear shiny red lips. Or if you wear black glasses, a strong smoke-eye makeup will look too "crowded" along with the black frames. If you wear very light, transparent frames, you can play with

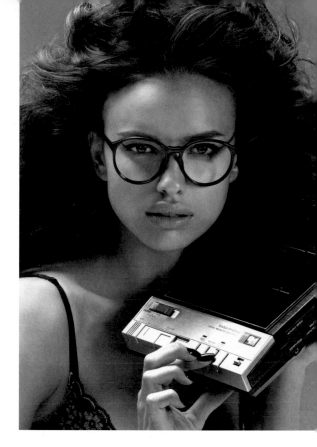

shadows more, because the frames won't be dominating your face. I did a classy black liquid eyeliner on Irina's eyes that goes well with her round-shaped frames. The makeup is very graphic and simple, and it doesn't look overdone. With strong red lips, the look would be too much.

*TIP* *Keep a cream-powder compact with you all the time to fix your makeup on the areas where the frame touches the skin.*

*If you wear extremely strong plus-vision glasses, your eyes will appear bigger. In that case you should apply black or dark-colored kohl inside the rims to make your eyes look smaller. Even light smoky eyes will "shrink" the eyes.*

*Minus-vision glasses make the eyes look smaller, so you can make them look bigger with a white kohl inside the rim and/or add darker eye shadow on the upper lash line and on the outer corners of your bottom lash line (to one-third of the length of the bottom lash line). Curling your lashes and using black mascara will also open up the eyes.*

## EVENING LOOK

Add a little transparent or ivory shimmer on the inner corners of your eyes to reflect light and give the illusion of bigger eyes. And remember that the style, material, and color of your frames should determine what kind of makeup you use. You don't need to get stuck with one style. Try different makeups. Find a balance that you feel comfortable with.

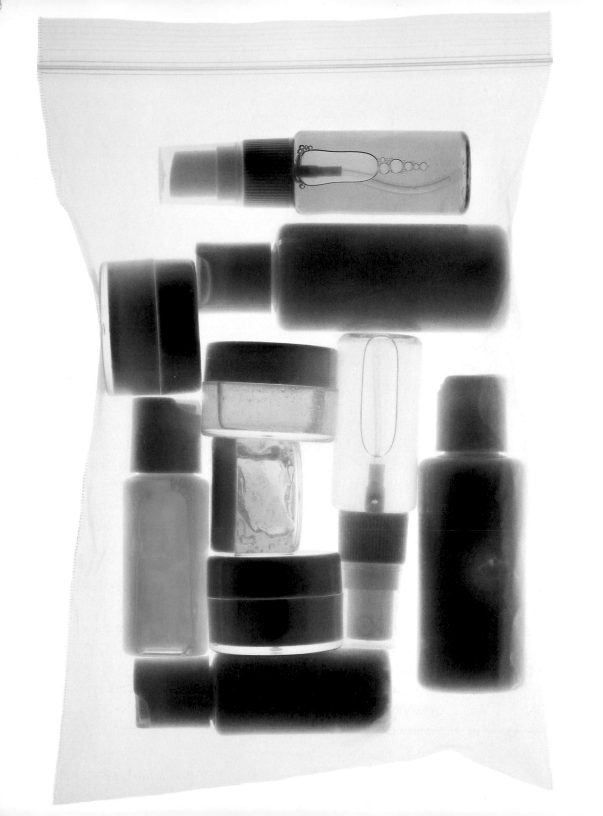

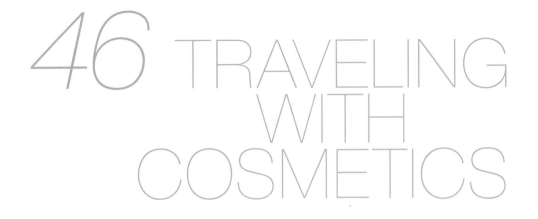

# 46 TRAVELING WITH COSMETICS

Do you remember when traveling with all your face creams and toners was as easy as stepping onto a bus? At least you didn't have to spend so much time thinking how to pack all your most important skin care and makeup products into a small ziplock bag! I have traveled with my makeup and skin care bags for the past twenty-two years, and I honestly consider myself a professional packer. And being a cosmetics junkie, I actually enjoy packing and transferring my creams and toners into travel-size containers. Small things can give great pleasure!

The whole process is not that complicated when you know a couple of facts before you hit the airport.

Flight time: Are you flying in the morning, midday, or late afternoon, or is the flight a red-eye? What is the duration of the flight?

- On a one-to-four-hour flight (short flight), you need only a lip balm to keep your lips moist and/or a small makeup kit (blotting papers, compact powder foundation, lip liner, lipstick or gloss).
- On a five-to-eight-hour flight (medium flight), take lip balm and makeup remover wipes that work like a hand sanitizer, refreshing your face as well as removing your makeup.

**SPRAY TONER:** Spray your skin type toner on your face every two hours in the lavatory to hydrate and freshen up. This feels really great on longer flights.

**FACE CREAM:** Apply to keep your face moist, especially on a red-eye.

**MAKEUP FOR A BUSINESS TRAVELER:** Compact powder foundation, a multistick that works for cheeks and lips and mascara.

**EXTRA TOOLS:** eyebrow pencil, lip pencil, eye pencil, makeup sponge, Q-tips. You can buy multipalette makeup collections at the airport tax free: minisize mascara, blush, eye shadows, brushes, and lipsticks in one handy case. Great for a business traveler.

• On a nine-to-fifteen-hour flight (long flight), your skin will need attention! Don't wear any makeup during such a long flight. Before the flight, apply a face serum and a thicker layer of your moisturizer. You can buy travel-size containers, into which you can transfer your creams and toners from your regular containers. Make sure the containers are no bigger than three ounces each.

## MUST-HAVE TRAVEL PRODUCTS

**SPRAY TONER.** Spray it on your face in the lavatory to get a small "shower" that really freshens up your skin and mood. Business and first-class lavatories carry some skin care products, including spray toners, but you should take your own. I carry an exfoliating cream that I use on my face three hours before landing. I love the feel, after 10 hours spent sitting and reading (and sometimes sleeping), of giving my face a minispa! I follow with a spray toner, then use a serum and a face cream. You can also buy travel-size skin care kits at the tax-free shop.

**EYE TREATMENT PADS.** Apply under your eyes for ten minutes. A moisturizing soft sheet face mask is a onetime face treatment: you just open the folded, moist sheet and apply it to your face for 15 minutes. It really moisturizes and is great for a superlong flight. (I use it on flights that are over 12 hours, and yes, you do look funny with a sheet on your face with holes cut out for your eyes, nose, and mouth.)

**HAND CREAM:** Great because you can massage your hands and arms with it and keep the blood circulation going!

**BUSINESS TRAVELERS:** You might need to pack skin care and makeup products in your cabin bag, in case you have to look fresh right after your flight and run for a meeting. It's best not to schedule a meeting immediately after a long flight, but if you have no choice, it's best to take your 9/11 makeup kit along: tinted moisturizer is the best choice, because the skin is drier than ever after a long flight. Just transfer the moisturizer to a smaller container. Concealer and loose powder finish the base. Don't try to do a very complicated eye makeup—just a black mascara and pencil liner. Blusher and lip makeup, and that's it!

A multistick might work for you as well. If you have a flight connection and have more than two hours between flights, have a massage, facial, and shower (many international airports offer these services nowadays) and do your makeup application right before the final flight. You will look fresher when finally landing at your destination.

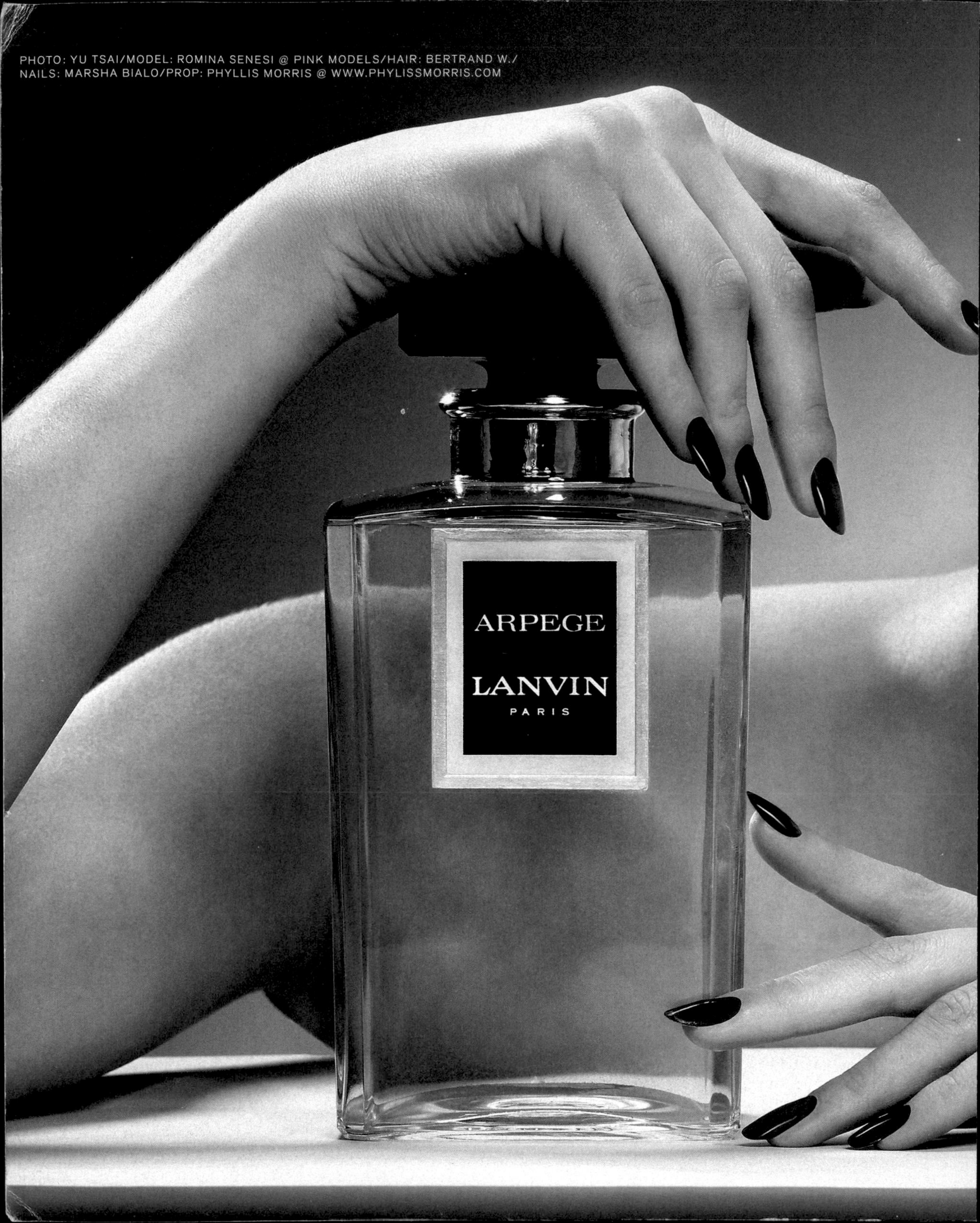
PHOTO: YU TSAI/MODEL: ROMINA SENESI @ PINK MODELS/HAIR: BERTRAND W./
NAILS: MARSHA BIALO/PROP: PHYLLIS MORRIS @ WWW.PHYLISSMORRIS.COM
ARPEGE
LANVIN
PARIS

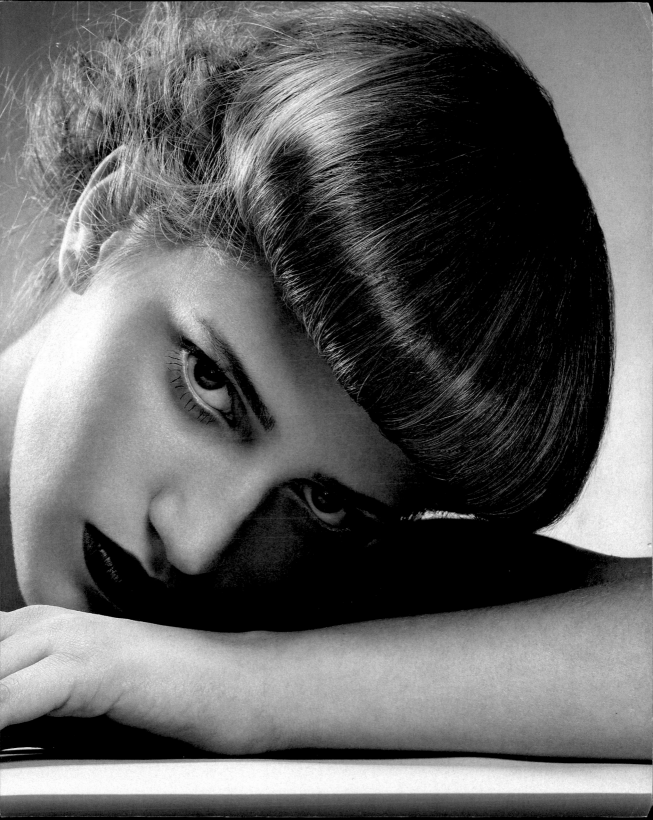

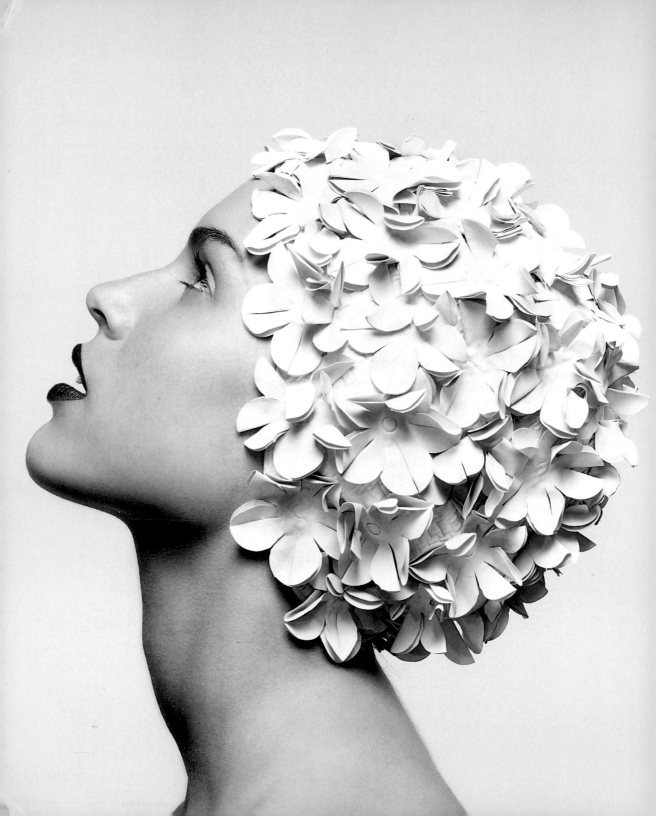

# THANK YOU

**This has been an amazing journey, and I want to thank all of you who have been involved with this publication. This book wouldn't be complete without your help. Thank you very much.**

First, I want to thank all the amazing artists and designers who have been inspiring me all these years and giving me the inspiration and motivation to keep me going: photographers, art directors, fashion designers, milliners, fashion stylists, hairstylists, and makeup artists whose art and creations have opened my eyes from my very early years until today.

Special thank you to Randee St. Nicholas. You are very special.

Photographers: Randee St. Nicholas, Daniela Federici, Nadia Pandolfo, Kemberly Marciano, Gitte Meldgaard, Cristina Trayfors, Kurt Iswarienko, Tony Duran, Yu Tsai, Warwick Saint, Giuliano Bekor, Nicolas Wagner, Colin Angus, Pascal Demeester, Evan Klanfer, Numi Nummelin, Kiino Villand.

A special thank you and big hugs to Jeffrey Gunthart @ www.rawcapturela .com for working on Kurt's and my images. You are the best!

All the models: thank you.

Thank you to my beautiful ladies: Lauren Hutton, Anne Archer, Lydia Hearst, Rebecca De Mornay, Shannen Doherty, Sunny Mabrey, and Alessandra Ambrosio.

Thank you actor Henry Ian Cusick and model/actor Jon Kotajarena.

Thank you Gary Mantoosh @ BWR Public Relations, Los Angeles.

A special thank-you to my friend Ole Henriksen, who helped me and opened my eyes, once again with the secrets of skin care.

Dr. Douglas Hamilton of Beverly Hills and eyebrow lady Gina Veltri at Byron & Tracey Salon Beverly Hills—thank you so much for sharing your beauty secrets!

Kathy Nenneker at the Los Angeles Times/Los Angeles Weddings.

Model agencies: Photogenics (thank you, Kemi and Nicole Bordeaux), LA Models (thank you, Monna, Anahid, and Andrew), IMG World (thank you, Peter), Elite Model Mgmt (thank you, Christopher, Philip, Jackie), Vision LA (thank you, Victor), One-Model Place (thank you, Jason), CESD (thank you, Alex and Stephanie), Ford (thank you, Gena), Marilyn NYC (thank you, Cheri), MC2 (thank you, Pink), Paparazzi (thank you, Laila), Next (thank you, Sarah and Jennifer), Industry Group (thank you, Jason), M4Models Hambourg (thank you, Tuomas), Click (thank you, Jamie).

Hairstylists: Bertrand W. at Tracey Mattingly, Keiko Hamaguchi at Celestine, Rob Talty at Magnet, Maranda at The Wall Group, Anthony Cristiano at Artists by Timothy Priano, Rodney Groves at Art Department, Kevin Woon at Jed Root, Gio Campora at The Wall Group, Yiotis at Celestine, David Keough at Celestine, Damian Monzillo at Aim Artists, Louise Moon at Sally Hershberger Salon, David Von Cannon at Bryan Bantry, Christian Marc at Celestine.

Fashion stylists: Heidi Meek at Cloutier, Martina Nilsson at Opus Beauty, Tim Bitici at Artists by Timothy Priano, Emma Trask, Leila Baboi, Petra Flannery at Margaret Maldonado, Vanessa Geldbach at Bryan Bantry.

Prop stylists: Amy Holland and Mathilda Christoffersen.

Nails: Beth Fricke at Artists by Timothy Priano for OPI, Jenna Hipp at Tracey Mattingly, Kimmie Keyes at Celestine, Marsha Bialo at Next Artists, and Libbie Simpkins.

A very special thank-you to Beth Fricke and OPI.

Thank you, Bobby Heller, Jorge Perez, and Ryan Supple at Opus Reps., Laura at Ray Brown, Megan and Sara at Creative 24, Mary Ellen Devaux at Randee St. Nicholas Studio, 88 Phases (Yu Tsai, Chalalai and the whole team), Kim Nabozny at Guess Inc., Scott Buccheit at Art Wing NY, Jared at Artists by Timothy Priano, retoucher Henry Kim at Big Lasso, Ed and Massimo at Smashbox Digital for retouchings.

A special thank you to Mr. Paul Marciano at GUESS, Inc.

My assistant Marco Souza.

A very special thank you to Sindee Campo whose artwork has been very inspirational to me all these years.

Thank you Lubov Azria at BCBGMaxAzria, Barney's New York, Marimekko.

A big hug to my supportive friends: Mindy Saad, Susanna Puisto, Nina Sallinen, Arya Kononen, Ulla Esposito, Laura Jappinen, Michelle Montes, Virpi Sidler, Juan-Carlos Escobar, Saimi Hoyer.

Thank you: L'Oréal USA: (Elizabeth Riley at Shu Uemura, Tim Quin at Armani Beauté, Erin at Lancôme) Nicole Blum at Guerlain, Make Up For Ever, Lumene at CVS & Kaplow Pr, Jamie at OPI.

Thank you Marita Tabermann-Coccaro and Ralph Coccaro at Taberco, Inc. for all your support. Love you guys!

Thank you, Exclusive Image Hollywood and Mr. Monet (www.imageexclusive.com).

Thank you Timothy Priano, all my agents and Christina and Ryan for PR at www.artistsbytimothypriano.com.

Special thank-you to Angelika Schubert and Anita Castillo at Celestine Agency. Thank you to my family for being there. A special thank-you to Kari Walden for being there when I really needed a supportive friend.

Special thank-you to Ann Song who put this book together with your magic touch.

Thank you, Malaika Adero, Todd Hunter, and Lisa Sciambra at Atria Books for your amazing work.

And finally a very special thank you to Judith Curr at Atria Books who believed in my vision and made this project happen.

Thank you Mikel Elliott at Smashbox and Quixote Studies, Los Angeles.

**SMASHBOX**

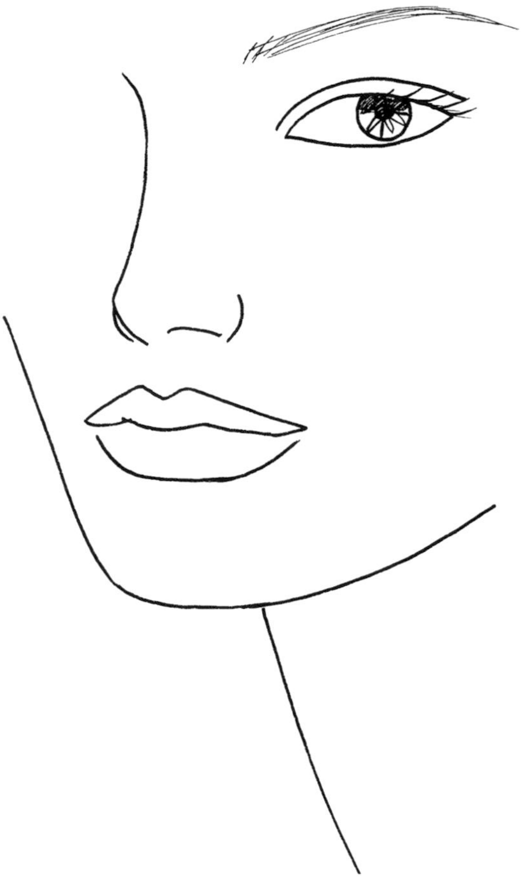

Skin care _____

_____

_____

_____

Concealer _____

_____

Foundation _____

_____

Powder _____

_____

Eyeshadow _____

_____

Eyeliner Pencil _____

_____

Liquid Liner _____

_____

Mascara _____

_____

Blush _____

_____

Lips _____

_____

Eyebrows _____

_____

Lipliner _____

_____

_____

_____

_____

_____

_____